Beating Mental Illness
My Five Steps to a Peaceful and Normal Life

克服心理疾病

让我获得平静正常生活的五个步骤

[美] 郝安迪 (Andy Hogan)　著

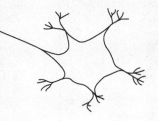

U0125716

中央民族大学出版社
China Minzu University Press

图书在版编目（CIP）数据

克服心理疾病：让我获得平静正常生活的五个步骤／
［美］郝安迪（Andy Hogan）著. —北京：中央民族大学
出版社，2018.6

ISBN 978-7-5660-1506-8

Ⅰ.①克… Ⅱ.①郝… Ⅲ.①心理疾病—防治—普及
读物 Ⅳ.①R395.2-49

中国版本图书馆 CIP 数据核字（2018）第 096504 号

克服心理疾病：让我获得平静正常生活的五个步骤

Beating Mental Illess

My Five steps to a Peaceful and Normal Life

作　　者　［美］郝安迪（Andy Hogan）
责任编辑　李苏幸
封面设计　舒刚卫
出 版 者　中央民族大学出版社
　　　　　北京市海淀区中关村南大街 27 号　邮编：100081
　　　　　电　话：68472815（发行部）传真：68932751（发行部）
　　　　　　　　　68932218（总编室）　　　68932447（办公室）
发 行 者　全国各地新华书店
印 刷 厂　北京建宏印刷有限公司
开　　本　787×1092（毫米）　1/16　印张：12.25
字　　数　200 千字
版　　次　2018 年 6 月第 1 版　2018 年 6 月第 1 次印刷
书　　号　ISBN 978-7-5660-1506-8
定　　价　62.00 元

内容简介

克服心理疾病：让我获得平静正常生活的五个步骤

郝安迪的著作就是他本人战胜过心理疾病并找到乐观，有好的结果甚至快乐生活的故事。第一章描绘出亲身经历躁郁症波涛般的内心激流。第二章到第六章描述五个步骤远离"心理疾病的激流"。步骤一的重点就是"察觉"真正症状的病因而看透所谓的表面症状。步骤二"承认"自己的疾病并不代表软弱或羞耻，反而表现着勇气以及负责任之心。步骤三"明白"疾病所带来的坏念头和习惯并不是病患个人的特质而是可以被治疗的症状而已。步骤四"控制"疾病的过程包括专业心理辅导，适当服药，以及培养健康关系。步骤五是设计并努力走向现实梦想而提升你的生活方式。

第七、第八章就是写给病患以及照顾他们的人的自助手册。

推　荐

北京工业大学人文社会科学学院法律系主任，一桥大学法学博士：张荆教授

中国目前有1600万重症的精神病人，还有大量的中轻度精神病患者，安迪的著作会对这些人和他们的家属有所帮助。该书是中英文对照本，对学英文的读者也有帮助。我尽力推荐！

Dr. Zhang Jing, Professor Dean, Beijing University of Technology

Currently there are 160 million people with severe mental illness in China, and a great number more who suffer from mental illness in lesser forms. Andy's book will be a great help to these people and their families. The book is in Chinese and English, so it can help those trying to improve their language skills as well. I whole-heartedly recommend this book!

瑞查·大卫森 MD，董事证明的心理医生

安迪在《克服心理疾病：让我获得平静正常生活的五个步骤》提到的五个步骤挺优秀的。这部简明易读的著作来自一位"有经验"的人。有时候小事情也可以很深刻。安迪的指教就是别人常忽略深刻的小事。我相信有心理疾病的病患以及他们的照顾者能从研读和遵从这些步骤的过程中而获益。

Richard S. Davidson MD, Board Certified Psychiatrist

The five steps Andy outlines in *Beating Mental Illness*; *My Five Steps to a Peaceful and Normal Life* are excellent. They are presented in clear, down-to-earth language from one who has "been there." Small things are often profound. Andy's book gives practical advice regarding small things often overlooked by others. I believe people with bipolar disorder, as well as their caregivers, can benefit greatly from reading and following them.

NAMI 犹他州（全美心理疾病联盟）

　　您读完此书最后一页之前，郝安迪已经成为您的儿子或兄弟了。他精彩和幽默的写法使得此书易看易懂。读者会很难忘安迪是如何度过躁狂症事件的。虽然安迪现在已经康复了，但他一辈子都会受这一疾病的影响，他感人至深的这本书证明了心理疾病是可以治疗的，而且病患者还能找到有意义的生活。

NAMI Utah（National Alliance for the Mentally Ill）

Long before you have reached the final page, Andy Hogan has become your son or your brother. His eloquent writing skills and his sense of humor make this book very readable. The reader will hardly forget the anguish and horrors Andy's book describes both from his recollections and from those who were present during the episodes. Even after recovery, Andy's life will remain overshadowed by his illness, but as his impressive book proves, a meaningful life can be found because mental illnesses are medically treatable.

目　录

Table of Contents

前　言

人们对于心理疾病的了解，应当说还处于初级阶段。虽然如此，在过去的十几年中，人们通过医生、社工以及其他心理专家出版的著作，对心理疾病的了解有了很大的进步。不过在心理疾病的教育过程中一直缺少一部重要的著作，那就是病患本人战胜心理疾病并找到方法，乐观、有好结果甚至快乐生活的故事。

我就是这样的人。我叫郝安迪，而我二十多年前被诊断为精神病，更准确地说是抑郁躁狂症或躁郁症。我从小就有抑郁以及躁狂的症状。经过好多年的痛苦（这痛苦并不只是我自己的，我的家庭和朋友们也因我的疾病而受了苦），我才察觉、承认、明白和控制自己的疾病，从而提升生活方式。

Preface

Understanding of mental illness is still in the elementary stages. Great strides forward have been made over the last decade as publications from doctors, counselors, and other medical professionals have come available. Still, there has always been one lacking element desperately needed in the education process: the personal triumph stories from those with the illness who have found a way to live positive, productive, and even pleasurable lives.

I am such a person. My name is Andy Hogan and I have been diagnosed with mental illness, specifically bipolar disorder, for over 20 years. I have had symptoms of depression and mania since childhood. It took many years and a lot of heartache, not just to myself but also to my family and friends, to discover and move through the process of identifying, authorizing, understanding, and controlling my illness, and then living a heightened life where dreams could once again come true.

我相信学习和遵从这五个步骤可以帮助您或您所爱的心理疾病的病患者找到更平静的生活，回归正常生活状态。我希望与您分享这些步骤可以让您很快地发现，虽然我自己患了严重精神病的一种，但还能学会过好生活，那么您或您所爱的病患者也可以。

我的这本书的后面还包含一个自助手册。手册的第一部分是写给抑郁躁狂症患者的。第二部分是写给病患的家人、朋友还有照顾者。这些手册提供活动，启发思想的疑问，还留有空白地方写日记。

I believe learning about and following these five steps can help you or your mentally ill loved one to find a more peaceful and normal life. I hope that sharing these steps with you can help you quickly realize, if I can find a good life despite my chronic mental illness, you or your loved one can too.

I have also included a self-help workbook which comes in two sections; one for those suffering from bipolar disorder, and one for their friends, family, and caregivers. These workbooks provide you with activities, thought - provoking questions, and areas for journaling.

第一章　远离心理疾病激流的五个步骤

当我的志愿服务领导者肯特抵达中国台湾的潮州镇（屏东）时，情况已经很棘手了。他一接到我的同事惊慌的电话：“我们不知道怎么回事，安迪突然疯了！”便立即开车由台中南下。当时没有任何一个人——包括我自己在内——知道我得了严重抑郁躁狂症（心理疾病的某种）！几年后，肯特告诉我，当他抵达潮州找到我的时候，我“看起来好像刚跟人打过架 —— 头发凌乱、衣衫不整、全身汗湿、慌乱又激动，而且精疲力竭”。肯特说当时的情形让他感到震惊惶恐：他试着和我说话，但我没有回答，反而哭了起来，跪在他面前，想亲吻他的双脚。

Chapter 1　Five Steps Out of the
Mental Illness Rapids

The situation was desperate when my volunteer service leader, Kent, finally arrived at the scene in Chao Chou, Chinese Taiwan. He had immediately driven down from Taichung following a frantic phone call from my colleagues stating that, "We don't know what's wrong; Andy just flipped out." No one, including myself, knew I was suffering a bipolar (a type of mental illness), manic psychosis episode. Kent later told me, that when he got to Chao Chou he found me, "looking like you had been in a fight - completely disheveled, sweat soaked, rumpled, flushed, and out of gas." Kent said it was shocking and frightening. He tried to talk to me. Instead of responding, I burst into tears, fell down on my knees before him, and tried to kiss his feet.

肯特见我的状况十分严重，便一口气冲到后面的房间，打电话给我在美国的父母。肯特告诉我父亲情形之后，才得知我母亲也有躁郁症病史；肯特立即安排我与一位在高雄凤山的心理医生午夜急诊。打完了电话，肯特请我那两位精疲力竭的同事——亚伦和麦克，把我弄上车。我相信他们一定很高兴终于可以离开，因为在他们努力照顾我的那几个小时里，我给了他们不少麻烦及折腾：我以为亚伦是耶稣基督，想好好拥抱他并亲吻他的脸；又以为麦克是魔鬼，尖叫着试图命令他离开。当他们想带我上车时，我还猛力去咬麦克的大腿，最后把我安顿在车子后座的中间位子上，他们分别坐在我的左右两边以防止更多问题发生。

Seeing the severity of the condition I was in, Kent rushed to the back room to make a phone call to my parents in America. He spoke with my dad, who informed him of my mother's history with manic-depressive, or bipolar disorder. Kent also set up a late night, emergency visit with a psychiatric doctor in the neighboring city of Feng Shan. After finishing his phone calls, Kent told my frazzled colleagues, Aaron and Mike, to get me in the car. I'm sure they were grateful to be leaving. While trying to contain me for the past several hours, I had put Aaron and Mike through everything from extended hugs and kisses when I thought Aaron was Christ, to attempts at casting Mike out when I became convinced he was Satan. As they tried to pull me into the car I bit Mike's leg as hard as I could. They finally got me into the middle of the back seat. There they could sit on both sides of me and try to prevent other problems.

午夜时分，我们抵达了凤山，罗医生已在那儿等着我们。他问了我一些问题，例如："What is your name? Where are you? Is it nighttime or day?（你叫什么名字？你在什么地方？现在是晚上还是白天？）"我无法回答他的问题，因为当时我心里只想搞清楚：究竟一个华人跟我说英语有何深刻意义和结果？当罗医生与我说话时，麦克卷起他的长裤，查看我在他腿上咬出的伤：紫黑色而且还流着血的一圈齿痕。于是麦克离开病房，请一位护士替他包扎伤口。回来的时候，有个强壮的护士（麦克的日记里写着她足足有300多磅）和他一起回到病房，看到那护士，我的头脑中随即响起一个声音命令我说："你必须娶那女人为妻！"在惊惧中，我大声尖叫着跳起来并试着逃跑。他们想抓住我时，我狠狠地对他们又踢又抓，最后他们三人一起抓我才没有让我跑掉。

We arrived in Feng Shan around midnight. Dr. Luo was waiting. He asked me some questions like, "What is your name? Where are you? Is it nighttime or day?" I couldn't answer because my mind was too boggled trying to figure out the deep meaning and eternal consequences of a Chinese person speaking to me in English. While Dr. Luo spoke to me, Mike rolled up his pants to look at his leg where I had bitten him. There was a dark purple and black mouth mark that was still bleeding. He left the room to ask a nurse for a bandage. When he returned, a very large nurse (300 pounds, as Mike recorded in his journal) followed him back. When I saw her, an impulse in my head commanded, "You must marry that woman!" In sheer terror, I screamed, jumped up, and tried to run away. When they tried to restrain me, I kicked and clawed viciously. It took all three together to keep me from fleeing.

他们把我按倒在地，麦克抓着我的一只手臂，亚伦抓着另一只手臂，肯特则压坐在我的肚子上。我激烈地前后摇晃着头，并用中英文大声地呼喊着，要耶稣基督来救我。

此时，罗医生给我打了一针——亚伦在日记中所说的"怪物镇静剂"，才让我好好地睡着——一睡就是好几天。他们把我带回车上，连夜开车到台北，以避开清晨拥挤的交通。虽然三位相关朋友的日记与回忆中都表示我过了一两天后就醒了，但我对此印象非常模糊。我记得的第一件事，就是在一间很小很暗的房间里醒来，脑中清醒的解放感犹如涸鱼归渊——我是那尾被捕上岸后又被放回水里的鱼。当时我睁开眼，一位陌生人坐在我床前，他看到我望着他时，微笑着对我说："我叫哈维，我是台北地区的志愿服务领导人。我会陪你直到肯特帮你办好一切手续并送你回家。"

They laid me on my back with Mike holding down one arm, Aaron the other, and Kent sitting on my middle. I started thrashing my head back and forth, screaming in English and Chinese for Jesus to save me. At that point, Dr. Luo gave me a "monster tranquilizer," as Aaron recorded in his journal, that finally put me to sleep – for several days. They carried me out to the car and drove through the night to avoid morning traffic in Taipei. Although the journals and memories of those involved all say I awoke after a day or so, my memories are very clouded. The first thing I remember is waking up in a bed in a very small and dark room. The relief of a sane mind felt as welcome as water to a "caught and released" fish. I opened my eyes and saw a strange man sitting on the bed. When he saw me looking at him, he smiled and said, "I'm Harvey, the service leader for Taipei. I'll be staying with you while Kent gets everything ready for you to go home."

我小声地"哦"了一声之后闭上眼睛，再次跌入深沉疲倦的睡眠之中。

接下来我只记得坐在机场里的一张四周围绕着花坛的长椅上。肯特手上拿着注射器及针筒对我说："我们只是要确定你能安全回到家。"我只麻木地点了点头让他们帮我打针。我记得有一位陌生人陪我走下一段狭窄的走廊（肯特的一位美国朋友刚好到台湾地区出差，便自告奋勇送我回美国）。当我再醒来时，人已在飞机上，坐在两个陌生人中间。其中一位手上拿着塑胶花盒，说："我们在台湾制造这些东西。"

我回答一声"哦"便又倒头睡着了。抵达旧金山时，我记得自己跑向父母亲，并拥抱他们。

Uttering a quiet "Oh," I closed my eyes and fell back into a deep and exhausted sleep. The next thing I remember is sitting on a bench that surrounded a planter at the airport. Kent, with a syringe and needle in his hand said, "We just want to make sure you get home without any incident." I numbly nodded and he gave me an injection. I remember walking down a narrow hallway escorted by a stranger. (A friend of Kent happened to be on a business trip in Taiwan. He volunteered to take me back to the States.) The next time I woke up, I was on a plane sitting between two strangers. One was holding plastic flower cases. "We have these manufactured in Taiwan. " the man said. "Oh. " I replied, and fell back to sleep. Arriving in San Francisco, I remember running up and hugging my parents.

我不明白为什么每次当我尝试和母亲交谈时，她总是回答我"我不会说中文，你得和我说英语。"我试着继续和她说话，但她还是听不懂。最后，只要我说完一句话，她便会说："I don't know, but I love you."（"我不懂你说什么，但是我爱你。"）

啊，真是一段不可思议的旅程！当我之前离开美国准备前往中国台湾时，我知道生活将会有所不同，但我万万没想到竟会变得如此天翻地覆。我怎能预料到当我返乡的时候，自己会亲身体验到"发疯"的真正感受。

去中国台湾之前，"疯子"只是年少时挖苦人的话，就像朋友告诉我他为他的宠物鱼取名亚力克时，我开玩笑地对他说："你真是个疯子！"当时纯粹是好笑，然而现在没人笑得出来了。

It was confusing that every time I tried to talk to my mom, she replied, "I don't speak Chinese. You have to speak in English." I kept trying to talk to her, but still she didn't understand. Finally, after everything I said, she would reply, "I don't know, but I love you."

Whoa. What a trip! When I left for Taiwan area, I knew my life was about to change. But I had no idea it would turn completely inside out. How could I have guessed I would return home knowing first-hand the answer to the question, "What is it like to go crazy?" Before Taiwan, "crazy" people were only the objects of my youthful sarcasm. "You must be a loony!" I said jokingly to my buddy when he told me he named his pet fish Erik. It was funny then. No one was laughing now. This was serious.

当时我没料到，打麻醉针半梦半醒由台湾飞回家的经历，只是我之后不断被躁郁症折磨的开始。在美国的普柔浮医院，有长达一个月的时间我不断地否认病情并掩饰抑郁。最后我的医生终于不情愿地让我出院，而我得以继续我的志愿服务。我被重新分配到蒙大拿州服务，那里的生活又湿又冷，抑郁症像一块巨大的冰块把我封在里面。那种不舒服的感觉不仅仅是悲伤难过，无论我做什么事或是去哪里，我的身体都感到焦虑不安，无法摆脱。我的思想窒息，精力冻结，甚至灵魂也感到冰冷，抑郁，死去……有时候，我一天中最大的成就，仅仅是能够从床上爬起来。

I didn't realize it at the time, but flying home from Taiwan in a tranquilized blur was only an introduction. From that point on, bipolar disorder would be my constant companion. After a month of desperate denial and masked depression in a Provo hospital, my doctor reluctantly gave the okay for me to leave the psychiatric ward and continue my volunteer service. Life in Montana, my reassigned area, started out clouded and cold. Depression became a giant ice cube I was trapped inside. The resulting discomfort was more than just sadness; it made me physically anxious and no matter where I went or what I did, I couldn't escape. It suffocated my mind and froze the energy inside my body. Even my spirit felt chilled, blue, and dying. Sometimes my biggest success of the day was just getting out of bed.

　　那段时期我所忍受的"精神寒冬"就像蒙大拿州一月的天空一样，是一片茫然无际的黑暗。时间流逝得很慢，但没有停止。两个月之后，仿佛番红花小心翼翼地在开始融雪的大地上悄然蔓延，我的热情也开始绽放，重新感到愉悦与自信。只可惜，这原来只是暴风雪在来临之前，刻意诱使小花绽放，使它接着遭受酷寒而冻死的一丝暖流。

　　原以为我的"抑郁病寒冬"已经过去了，所以不再吃药，结果不久，一场比在台湾地区更严重的"躁郁症龙卷风"袭来，让我进了蒙大拿州波兹曼市的医院。当我趴在病房的地板上像蛇一般匍匐爬行、臭骂医生时，医生对我的领导说："像他这样的病患通常要好几年才会恢复正常，有的人则一辈子都不会好。安迪很可能永远也不会像以前一样了。"

The mental winter I suffered at that time felt as vast as the dark, January, Montana sky. Time dragged, but didn't stop. Two months later, as the yellow crocus cautiously crept up from the thawing ground, my enthusiasm also began to blossom. I started feeling spry and confident again. Sadly, it turned out to be only the warm before the storm that tempts the buds to bloom only to die in a ferocious freeze. Thinking my bipolar winter had passed, I quit taking my medication. Soon, a manic tornado even more serious than the one in Taiwan blew me into a hospital in Bozeman. As I scooted around the examining room on my belly and hissed poisoned expletives at the doctor, he told my service leader, "People in this condition usually take years to recover. Some never do. Andy may never be the same again."

医生和护士在一阵激烈的手忙脚乱之后，他们终于决定给我打一剂强烈的镇静剂让我安静下来，直到隔天的傍晚我才醒来。我的父母已经搭飞机过来陪我了，但院方要到隔天早上才准我出院，这让我在监狱般的观察室中度过了痛苦的一晚，父亲陪我睡在又冷又硬的瓷砖地上。我则坐在一张薄垫子上，背靠着没有门把的门。数小时，我的眼睛盯着角落的不锈钢马桶、淡黄色的墙壁，以及天花板上的摄影机，心想着我能不能再恢复到正常的生活。我可以再度大笑，或者微笑吗？我可以再去跑马拉松，再到山上滑雪，再到河边钓鱼吗？我会遇到一位不怕我的"发疯"病史，或愿意下嫁精神病患的女子吗？如果结婚了，我可以工作养家吗？我的孩子会正常吗？

After an intense struggle with doctors and nurses, they finally resorted to a strong sedative injection to settle me down. I awoke just at nightfall the next day. My parents had flown in to be with me. The hospital wouldn't let me check out until morning. So, I spent a torturous night in the cell-like holding room. Dad slept next to me on the cold, hard tile. Unable to sleep, I sat on a thin pad with my back pressed against the locked, handle-less door. I stared for hours at the stainless steel toilet in the corner, the plain yellow walls, and the camera in the ceiling, wondering if my life could ever be normal again. Would I be able to laugh or even smile again? Would I ever run another marathon, ski another mountain, or fish another stream? Would I be able to find a girl who wouldn't be afraid of my *crazy* recent past or the thought of being married to a mentally ill person? If I did get married, could I ever hold a job and raise a family? Would my children be normal?

在强效药物造成不安和忧郁之下，这些思想像铅板一般击打着我的身心，我感到绝望、无助，彻底地被击垮。当时的我没有想到，这些问题的所有答案，竟然都同样是铿锵有力的一声："可以！"

自从躁郁症第一次把我抛向无止境的狂躁高塔和忧郁深渊的云霄飞车循环，至今为止，已足足有二十几年。回头想想，我知道当时在波兹曼的医生说的没错，只不过不是他所想象的那样——没错！的确需要花好几年才能恢复。没错！我已经不再是同一个人了。但那位医生没看见的是，"不再是同一个人"在我身上变成一件美好又神奇的事。躁郁症确实改变了我的人生，因为有了治疗它的经验，使我现在成为一位更好的人，就像熔炉的烈火把金矿中不洁的成分烧毁殆尽，留下最纯粹的黄金一样，这疾病也让我变成了一位被塑造过、精炼且更臻纯洁的人。

In my drug enhanced state of anxiety and depression, these thoughts felt like sheets of lead being thrown on my mind and body. I felt hopeless, helpless, and completely squashed. I never would have guessed the answer to each of these questions would be a resounding, "YES!" It's been well over a decade since the first time bipolar disorder threw me on the never-ending up and down roller coaster cycle. Looking back, I can see the doctor in Bozeman was right…but not in the way he was thinking. Yes, it took years to recover. Yes, I have never been the same again. The part the doctor didn't see was that "not ever being the same again" turned into a good and wonderful thing! It's true bipolar disorder changed me. Because of its demands, I am now a better person. Just like the refining fire burns out impurities from gold nuggets, so has this illness made me a molded, refined, and more pure person.

这些年来与慢性心理疾病的对抗，让我学习到许多只有患了此病才能体会到的事情。其中最大的收获，便是明白躁郁症虽然无法根治，但却是可以治疗的；换句话说，就是患病者仍有可能拥有一个有意义、有成就、丰富且快乐的人生！当年在波兹曼发病时，同事们十分慌张地开车送我去医院，在车上的我几乎用尽了意志力，才控制住自己不去打开车门，跳到对向的车阵中结束生命，结束一切。那时死亡似乎是唯一的逃避方法。然而现在每当我和儿子互丢水球，或和女儿一起跳弹力床的时候，看到他们眼中的温馨快乐与喜悦，便庆幸自己能选择活下来。每天晚上，我都与妻子跪下祈祷，感谢神又赐给我们充满祝福的一天。

Dealing with this chronic mental illness for all these years has taught me lessons I never would have learned without it. One of the greatest lessons I gained is the knowledge that bipolar disorder, though not yet curable, is highly treatable. In other words, it is still possible to live a purposeful, productive, and even pleasurable life! During my breakdown in Bozeman, as my colleagues frantically drove me to the hospital, it took all of my willpower to restrain myself from ending it all by opening the door and jumping out of the car into the oncoming traffic. Death seemed to be the only escape. Now, as I have water balloon wars with my son and bounce on the trampoline with my daughter, I see happiness and joy in the warm, glowing light of their eyes. Each night I kneel with my wife in prayer and thank God for another blessed day of life.

　　如何能从日复一日想自杀的抑郁及难以控制的躁狂循环中脱离，并进步到拥有稳定的人际关系与安定情绪的生活呢？说起来真不是一件容易的事。回顾我的过去种种，好像在看一部电影。第一幕，我看见自己在闪亮的生命之河上飞镖钓鱼，蜜蜂嗡嗡地叫着，鸟儿快乐地歌唱着，松林中有美妙的音乐回荡着。转瞬之间，当我刚钓起一尾精明的彩虹鳟鱼时，突然一个失足，跌进巨大的心理疾病激流和沮丧深渊里。这股激流绕着一座巨大石块盘旋不去。当我在激流中翻滚之际，我看见岩石上有文字深深刻着：

　　"我需要帮助，我有弱点，我愿意听别人的意见并改变我自己。"

　　这些字旋转着渗镂在巨石的表面，一如攀岩的凹槽，足以用手攀住来抵抗心理疾病的激流。

　　How is it possible to progress from a daily cycle of demonic depression and uncontrolled mania to a life of stable relationships and steady emotions? To say the least, it hasn't been easy. Looking back on my life is like watching a movie. In the opening scene, I picture myself fly fishing in the sparkling river of life. Bees are humming and sweet birds are singing. Music is ringing through the pines. Suddenly, right when I hook into a brilliant rainbow trout, I trip into the rapids of pounding mania and drowning depression. These rapids circle a giant boulder. As I roll in the rapids I can see the words: "I need help. I have weakness. I am willing to listen to others and change myself." carved deeply into the rock. The words spiral up the rock and can be used as handholds out of the mental illness rapids.

一开始，我没有心怀感恩地去理会那些凹槽，反而自大地拒绝借助这些简单的文字，让它们来帮助我，于是多年来，我像个筋疲力尽的笨蛋，不断地围绕着此一激流中的岩石跌跌撞撞；许多人想要伸手将我从心理疾病的激流中拯救出来，有些人甚至差一点连自己也被卷进激流。到最后，唯一能拯救我的方法，还是选择抓住巨石上的凹槽，靠着凹槽的助力爬上巨石。当我爬到最高处时我看到更多的刻字："恭喜你！你找到了谦卑之石！"

我从"谦卑之石"上俯瞰整条河流，看见我所爱的人们站在远处，正用手指着能引领我远离心理疾病激流，走向平静之水的五块清晰的踏脚石。

Instead of accepting the handholds with gratitude, I arrogantly refuse to grasp and benefit from these simple words. Like a ragged rascal, for years I stumble and tumble round and around that rugged rock. Many helping hands try to pull me out of the mental illness rapids. Some of them almost get sucked in themselves. In the end, the only thing that can save me is choosing to take hold of the handholds, and with great effort use them to climb up the giant boulder. Standing on top, I see more words carved in the rock. They read, "Congratulations, You Have Found Rock Humility." From the top of Rock Humility, I look out over the river and see distant loved ones pointing to five distinct stepping-stones leading through the mental illness rapids toward more peaceful waters.

　　每一块踏脚石上也都有刻字。第一块刻着"察觉",第二块是"承认",第三块是"明白",第四块是"控制",第五块则是"提升";每一块踏脚石都是通往下一块的必经之地。我一块接一块跳上这些踏脚石,终于找到脱离奔腾激流的途径,走入比较平静且能掌握的水流,当我停下来头不再旋转时,我发现先前钓上来的大鳟鱼,仍然钩在我的鱼竿上——这部电影就在我"转向"积极、有工作能力且正常的生活时终于落幕。虽然至今躁郁激流仍在我生命中激起大小浪花,但现在我已知道如何掌握它们。在那些较缓和的激流里,我已可以回头查看过往的心理疾病激流,知道自己并不孤单。有许多人也正被卷入躁郁症或其他心理疾病的高低摆盪之激流。

　　There are words carved in each stepping stone. The first reads, "Identify;" the second, "Authorize;" the third, "Understand;" the fourth, "Control;" and the fifth, "Heighten." Each stone is necessary to reach the next. One by one, I jump to each stone and eventually find my way out of the rushing rapids and into more peaceful and manageable waters. As my head stops spinning, I realize the trophy trout I had originally hooked is still on my line. The movie comes to an end as I reel in a positive, productive, and normal life. The waters I ended up in still splash highs and lows into my life, however, now they are manageable. In these more peaceful waters, I'm able to look back at the mental illness rapids I have navigated and see that I wasn't alone. There are many others spinning, spiraling, and often being sucked under in the cyclonic highs and lows of bipolar disorder or other mental illnesses.

在我看到水中有些人只为了生存的一口气而挣扎搏斗时，我也同时看到他们的亲人及好友们走进深不可测且瞬息万变的水流里，冒着极大的危险，试图想要拯救他们；然而这些亲友们虽然怀着真诚的热情，却不知道该做什么或怎么帮忙，于是他们经常挫败，认为心理疾病激流的威力太过强大，"拯救任务"的完成根本是不可能的事。

所以，为了那些卷入激流中的人，以及那些试图帮助他们的人，我想要传递一个希望的讯息：我已找到勘查激流的方法，愿意将我发现的途径绘成图，装入防水的玻璃瓶中，抛入生命之河来传播这个讯息。我知道这小小的"瓶中信"无法拯救所有的人，但是我相信它一定可以帮助很多人。

As I watch them battle for the simple breath of life, I can also see multitudes of loved ones and caregivers wading into the deep and treacherous water, risking much while trying to save them. Many of these would−be rescuers, though sincere in their desires, don't know what to do or how to help. Too often they retreat in defeat, thinking the rapids are too powerful and the "saving mission" is impossible. To both those caught in the rapids and those wishing to find a way to help, I want to send out a message of hope. Now that I've found a way to navigate the mental illness rapids, I wish to map out the path I found, stuff it in a watertight bottle, and cast it out into the river of life. I know my little "message in a bottle" isn't the solution for everyone. But, I do believe it can help many.

　　想象一下：一个被困在激流之中的人，要看见装在瓶中的讯息是多么困难的事。但如果那个人能在激流中，找到并爬上一块大岩石呢？他获救的机会就很大了！这块大岩石就是我所说的"谦卑之石"。它静立在高耸之处，使卷入激流中的人能轻易地看见、攀登，并能在这块大石上清楚地看见我放在水中的"瓶中信"，从而了解到蕴藏于我所说的五个步骤之中的真理。一旦登上了"谦卑之石"，还可以让他们有最大的机会看到并踏上"察觉"之石——就是我所谓的心理疾病激流之五块踏脚石的第一块巨石。

　　Think how hard it would be to find and read a message in a bottle while drowning in rapids. It would be practically impossible. But what if the people could find and climb a giant stone in the middle of the rapids? Their chances would greatly improve. Rock Humility provides a lofty perch where people caught in the rapids can more easily spot my "message in a bottle," and see truth in the steps outlined inside. Starting from Rock Humility will also give them the greatest chance to see and reach "Identify," the first of the five stepping-stones out of the mental illness rapids.

第二章　步骤一：察觉你的疾病

正常的头脑知道它没病

生病的头脑认为它没病

现在我来谈谈自己被诊断的心理疾病。在美国，有 200 万以上的人饱受躁郁症折磨，还有许多人未被发现，或被误诊为其他病情，因此实际上患病者的人数可能比此数据多一倍！为什么这种疾病那么难以察觉？我相信原因有很多，其中原因或许是这种病的症状往往要到了成人时才变得严重。另一个可能的理由则是，每一个人都会有些不同程度的抑郁或躁狂症状。事实上，当你读了这本书之后，会毫不犹豫地自问："我也有不少甚至是所有的这些症状！我患了躁郁症吗？"请永远记得，躁郁症会将这些或多或少的症状——原本是正常的情绪反应——推向极端严重的情况，而发作时的严重程度也因人而异。

Chapter 2 Step One: Identify Your Illness

A normal mind knows it isn't ill

An ill mind thinks it isn't ill

Let's talk about my specific, diagnosed mental illness. Over 2,000,000 people in America suffer from bipolar disorder. This number could be double because so many are either undiagnosed or misdiagnosed. Why is this disorder so tough to identify? I'm sure there are many reasons. One reason could be that the symptoms often don't go to the extreme until early adulthood. Another could be because everyone experiences depression and mania in varying degrees. In fact, as you read this book, you will undoubtedly say to yourself, "I have many or all of these symptoms! Do I have bipolar disorder?" Always remember, bipolar disorder pushes symptoms *to the extreme*. These extremes vary with each individual.

发现躁郁症的要诀是：察觉在什么情况下自己或亲人的情绪会显得异常高昂或低落。所谓“正常”其实是一个很难拿捏的词，因为每个人的“正常”情形都不一样。当你很了解一个人时，在状况发生时，你一定能发觉哪儿不对劲，我认为躁郁症之所以难以察觉的最大原因之一，是因为人们不愿意好好地去认识一个人。如果我们妄下断语说“她只是个疯子”，或我们不假思索地说“她只要想清楚了就好”，或我们没有看清事实，便轻松地做出“其实这根本没有问题”之类的判断，我们怎么能去了解一个人呢？就是因为秉承这种“无知的傲慢”心态来与他人相处，让我无法趁早学到该如何在生活中察觉出躁郁症状，以下让我来解释为什么。

The trick to identifying bipolar disorder is to recognize when you or a loved one goes beyond normal highs and normal lows. “Normal” is a tricky word because it's different for everyone. When you know a person well, however, you recognize when something isn't right. I think one of the biggest reasons bipolar disorder too often goes unidentified is because of an unwillingness to know others well. How can we know a person well if we are quick to conclude, “She's just a loony；” if we automatically assume, “She just needs to snap out of it；” or if we turn our backs on reality with the cutting comment, “There's really nothing wrong.” Treating another with this attitude of “arrogant ignorance” turned out to be the very thing that kept me from knowing how to identify bipolar disorder earlier in my own life. Let me explain.

我应该可以从青少年时期的一个深夜，被父母房间里的尖叫声把我从平静的睡眠中吵醒的那一刻起，便开始学习如何察觉躁郁症的症状。当时我不知道到底发生了什么事情，于是偷偷走到他们的房门前，看见我父亲急切地想着要知道我母亲怎么了——我的母亲眼中露着惊惶，胡言乱语，大叫大喊着天使、号角和恶鬼。父亲完全不知道母亲是极度躁狂的病情发作，他以为她是被恶灵附身，因此一直试着想用祈祷将恶灵驱逐出去。几分钟后，祖父赶到我们家想要帮忙，母亲便尖叫着："他来了！他来了！恶鬼来了！把他赶出去！"我的父亲和祖父花了很久的时间才搞清楚母亲是精神病发作，而不是被魔鬼附身。终于他们做了正确的决定：送她到医院去。

I could have begun my education of how to identify bipolar disorder early in my teen years when late one night yelling in my parents' room awoke me from my peaceful slumber. Completely unaware of what was happening I sneaked to their bedroom doorway and spied as my dad tried desperately to figure out what was wrong with my mother. She had panic in her eyes and was shouting nonsense words about angels, trumpets, and ghosts. My dad had no idea she was suffering an extreme, bipolar manic episode. He thought she was possessed with an evil spirit and tried to use prayer to cast the demon away. A few minutes later when Grandpa arrived at our house to try and help, my mother yelled out, "There he is! The ghost! Cast him away!" It took a long time for Dad and Grandpa to realize she was mentally ill and not possessed. Finally, they did the right thing and took her to the hospital.

几个星期后，母亲出院回家。虽然她的发作病情已经过去，然而离康复遥遥无期。每天我看到她躺在沙发上，一个小时又一个小时哭哭啼啼地研读哲理书或哼歌令我厌烦至极。父亲下班回家时，母亲会对他诉说她是一个如何失败的妻子和母亲，邪恶的世界如何抢走她的家庭，还有她的寂寞、绝望与无助之感。有时晚上，当她的情绪从抑郁再度转变成躁狂时，母亲会把父亲拉到他们房间，持续好几个小时告诉他那些在她脑中缠绕不去的种种幻想，往往她的幻想会让她兴奋、激动起来，她会像路边候选人一样大喊大叫；虽然他们的房门关着，我们这些小孩总是要到母亲安静下来之后才得以入眠。

Mother came home after a few weeks in the hospital. Although the episode had passed, she was far from cured. Every day I watched in disgust as she slumped on the couch, reading philosophy books or humming songs, all the while crying and crying, hour after hour. When Dad came home from work, she would talk to him about her depressing failures as a wife and mother, how evil was out to get her family, and how alone, hopeless, and helpless she felt. Sometimes at night, when the depression cycled to mania, Mother would take Dad into their room and talk for hours about themes her mind had become obsessed on. She would often get so worked up by what she was saying that she would start yelling like a roadside preacher. Even though their door was closed, we children were unable to sleep until she quieted down.

我们这些孩子，当时只能靠自己来察觉母亲的问题，因为没有人真的了解她的病情，所以没有人为我们做任何说明。那时的我做了错误且幼稚的推论：我认为母亲的问题都只是她的脑袋在作祟，因为她太想要当个好人（甚至是圣人），而且花太多力气去了解一些哲理的事。那时候的我确信，如果她愿意放轻松、不想那么多，离开沙发做点运动，或者只是起身做点任何事情——除了哼歌及看书以外——的话，她就会感觉好过些。我完全不知道，当我告诉母亲这些意见的时候，就形同跟一个断了腿的人说："你只要起来走路就能解决问题了！"母亲的问题不是全在她的脑袋，而是跟断掉的腿骨一样，是需要被治疗的生理问题。一位老师绝不会对糖尿病正发作的学生说："别装病了，快去看书！你只需要调整你的态度！"

As children we were left to ourselves to identify Mother's problem. No one ever explained what was wrong because no one really knew. My erroneous, adolescent theory was that it was all in her head. I thought it was her own fault for being too "goodie-goodie" and trying too hard to understand philosophical things. I was sure if she would just chill out, stop thinking so much, get up off the couch and exercise, or just get up and do something besides hum songs and read books, she would feel better. I didn't realize when I told her this, it was the equivalent of telling someone with a broken leg just getting up and walking would solve his or her problem. Mother's problem was not "all in her head." Just like a broken bone, it was a physical deficiency in her body that needed treatment. A teacher wouldn't say to a student who was suffering from a diabetic attack, "Snap out of it and get to work! You just need an attitude adjustment."

不，老师会慈祥且尽快地为生病的学生找到需要的食物及药物。我母亲的抑郁和躁狂，其实就跟患糖尿病的学生发病没有两样。当时的她最需要的是家人的爱和了解，而不是残酷的批评和蔑视。假如当时我们全家一起坐下来，公开且坦诚地谈谈心中的感觉，以及讨论现实情况的话，可能会帮助我改变我的态度；可惜那时候，关于如何面对这种病的知识，就跟我妈尝试的药物一样新。如果那时候我选择表达更宽容的爱，并以"我相信你生病了"的包容态度来面对母亲，而不是用那种"你活该"的态度的话，我就会从真实生活中开始学习关于"躁郁症"的课程了。我不仅能学习到该如何帮助母亲从疾病中获得安慰，更可以帮助我自己早点获得在判断躁郁症时应有的经验与知识。

No, the teacher would kindly and quickly get proper food or medication for the student. My mother's depression and mania were no different than the diabetic student. The thing she needed most from her family was love and understanding, not cruel criticism and degrading disgust. I think it would have helped my attitude if, as a family, we could have talked about our feelings and the situation openly. But at that time, understanding of how to deal with the illness was as new as the medications my mother was trying. If I would have chosen to show greater love and accepted an attitude of "I believe you are ill," instead of, "You brought this upon yourself," I could have become a student in the real-life classroom of bipolar disorder. There I would have gained an education not only to help comfort my mother in her suffering, but also to give me the experience and knowledge I needed to identify the bipolar disorder in me earlier.

当时自私的我不但没有付出爱心去学习这些，反而吊儿郎当地选择忽略我的母亲。我用这种傲慢无知的心态看待母亲和她所得的病，就像把戴上焊接镜当作是太阳眼镜一样，大摇大摆地走在街头，还觉得自己好酷。你可以说当时的我简直就跟蝙蝠一样盲目。没有被发觉的躁郁症就跟吸血蝙蝠一样会欺骗人——人们一开始可能会误以为吸血蝙蝠是没有危险性的小老鼠，然而一旦被咬了，不幸的受害者就会毫不自觉地按照已生病（却不自知）的脑袋中所产生的念头和冲动去行动。然而，你不可能一辈子把十字架挡在面前过日子！那么你究竟该如何避免被"躁郁吸血鬼"咬上一口？答案就是在被抓进它黑暗的巢穴之前，先察觉敌人的存在。目前医学上还无法透过验血查出脑内引发躁郁症的化学成分不平衡问题，唯有从它引发的症状来辨识躁郁症。

Instead of lovingly seeking this education, I selfishly chose to play hooky and avoided my mother altogether. Viewing my mother and her illness with this attitude of arrogant ignorance was like wearing a welding hood as shades and strutting down teen-street thinking I was cool. You could say, at that time, I was pretty much "blind as a bat." Unidentified bipolar disorder is as deceiving as a vampire bat. At first, people view it to be a harmless house mouse. Then, when it bites, the unfortunate victim becomes oblivious to his or her condition and acts according to the whims and impulses of a sick mind. You can't go through life holding a cross in front of you. So how do you prepare for and avoid draco-polar's bite? The answer is to identify the enemy before it drags you into the extremes of its cave. Since there is no blood test to identify chemical imbalances in the brain, you have to recognize bipolar disorder from its symptoms.

就像世上没有两个人是完全一样的，每位躁郁症患者的症状也都因人而异。我个人把躁郁症引发的初期行为、言语及思想称为“表面症状”，此一症状在躁郁症还深藏不露的时候，最显而易见。要真正地察觉躁郁症，你必须看到表面症状以外的最终病因。例如在我母亲三更半夜大声对我父亲大喊一堆哲理时，如果具备足够的经验和知识，我不会误以为她是个烂好人或是太过于管制的人，反而能正确地判断造成她这些行为的根本原因，乃是她的躁狂症正在发作。我不会把母亲整天赖在沙发上哭哭啼啼当作是懒惰鬼的行为，而是能深入察觉真正的原因：化学成分不平衡造成的抑郁症。

Just as no two people are exactly the same, bipolar disorder's symptoms are also very individual – on the surface. I call the initial actions, words, and thoughts stemming from the disorder "surface symptoms." Surface symptoms are the obvious things you see while the deeper, underlying force remains hidden. The trick to identifying this devious bipolar disorder is to look beyond the surface symptoms and see the ultimate cause. For example, rather than mistaking the surface symptoms of my mother as "goodie-goodie" and "preachy" when she yelled philosophies at my dad in the middle of the night, experience and knowledge of the disorder could have helped me to correctly identify the real source: mania. Instead of seeing the surface symptom of a slacker crying on the couch all day, I could have looked deeper and identified the true symptom: out of balance, chemical depression.

其他一般躁郁症病人常有的表面症状还包括：太兴奋或太热衷于工作，以至于不安排时间吃饭或休息；在创作艺术上过于热情；极端的哲理狂热；随便乱花钱；在凌晨三点打电话给某个兄弟，讲一堆"超级好玩"的度假计划……这些都可能是躁狂症引发的表面症状。另一些极端的现象是，酒鬼嗜睡者，一天到晚迟到的员工，或者是在派对中不笑不跳舞，甚至话也很少的扫兴家伙；这些人都有抑郁症的倾向。躁郁症患者因为个性、年龄、性别及成长环境的不同，每个患者的表面症状也都各自不同。然而当你真正了解缘由时，你会发现这些症状都是起源于躁狂或抑郁。

Other surface symptoms common with bipolar disorder victims could include: being overly excited and enthusiastic about work – to the point of not taking time to eat or relax, creating art with over–zealous passion, over–the–top philosophical fanaticism, spending money frivolously, and even calling a brother at 3: 00 AM with ideas and plans for a "super–fun" vacation. In the extreme, all of these examples could be surface symptoms of bipolar mania. At the other extreme, you can have an alcoholic, someone who oversleeps every day, a chronically late employee, or even the "party pooper" who doesn't laugh, dance, or even talk much. These could all be people suffering from bipolar depression. With the millions of personality, age, gender, and upbringing differences, the surface symptoms people with bipolar disorder show appear to all be different. When you understand the source, however, you discover they are stemmed from either mania or depression.

　　这些症状的真正病因若能越早被正确地察觉及治疗，它们就越少有机会把日后生活搞得天翻地覆。为了提供你在"察觉"过程中的协助，我愿意在此分享及解释我个人在发病初期的表面症状。让我们来谈谈躁狂症的部分吧。在我即将成为青少年的时候，躁狂症就开始影响我的行为。某天晚上，我睡不着，站在床上往窗外看，研究夜空中的星星，开始思考"这些星星离地球有多远?"这些思考触发我不断想着宇宙的无穷无尽，更进一步引导我去思索人死后的事。我一向被教导，当我死后经过一段时间，我的身体跟灵体终会再次结合，及所谓的"复活"，复活之后我就会永远活下去。

　　当时的我想不透永恒究竟有多久，一股难以抗拒的思想奔驰，我感到四周的黑暗和无尽宇宙的重量像是直接压迫着我的心与胃。

The sooner these true sources can be correctly identified and treated, the less chance they have of developing into life-shattering extremes. Let me share and explain some of my own early surface symptoms to help in the identifying process. Let's talk about mania first. Mania started influencing my behavior in late childhood. One night I couldn't sleep. As I stood on my bedlooking out the window studying the nighttime stars, I started thinking about how far away they were. This sparked thoughts about the endlessness of the universe. This led to thoughts of life after death. I had been taught that after I died, eventually my body and spirit would come back together, and this was called resurrection. After the resurrection, I would live forever. As I failed to comprehend how long forever was, I felt overwhelmed. The surrounding darkness and weight of an endless universe seemed to press down on my heart and stomach.

我不知道该怎么做，或该怎么停止这些在脑海中打转的念头，所以我感到恐慌，觉得自己快疯了，最后我拖着脚步穿过大厅，眼中带泪地走进我父母的房间叫醒他们，大喊着"我们永远不会死！"之类的话。在我向被吓醒的父母解释我脑中的情况后，我记得父亲慈爱地回应我："像你这么年纪小的孩子怎么会在半夜想这么深奥的事？来吧，跟我们一起躺下来。"母亲在一旁轻轻按摩着我的背，他们一面和我说话，告诉我在今生有一些事情是我们无法了解的。事实上，他们的话没有什么作用，但是他们温暖的床、轻柔的触碰、在我耳边说他们爱我的话确实安慰了我，于是我很快地睡着了。像这种因"想太多而睡不着"的表面症状，似乎靠着一夜好眠就可以解决。当时没有人理解到那未被察觉的躁狂症已继续在我体内变化壮大。

I didn't know what to do or how to stop thinking about it. I started to panic and I felt like I was going crazy. Finally, I trudged across the hall in tears into my parents' room, woke them up, and burst out with something like, "We're never going to die!" After I explained myself to my startled parents, I remember my dad lovingly responding, "What is a young boy your age doing thinking about a deep subject like this in the middle of the night? Come lie down with us." My mother rubbed my back as we talked about it. They told me there are some things in this life that we just don't understand. Their words weren't comforting, but their warm bed, gentle touch, and soft voices were. Soon I fell asleep. The surface symptom of missing sleep due to deep thinking seemed to be easily fixed with a good night's rest. No one realized the true, unidentified mania continued mutating and multiplying inside me.

随着我渐渐成长，那些盘桓不去的躁狂思绪就像野火一样增生。看电影经常是这些思绪萌发的导火线。例如一次我正在棒球场上割草的时候，我的脑袋开始沉醉于迪士尼动画电影《阿拉丁》所传达的"潜意识讯息"，确信这部电影的制作人，不自觉地把秘密编入电影的情节里。要割完整座棒球场的草，通常要花上数小时，然而我当时因为被自己的奇想吞没，以至于完全没有注意到时间的流逝。割完草后，我兴致勃勃地和我的伙伴分享我脑中的想法，但他的反应却出乎我意料，一点都不觉得兴奋或感动，只说："这段时间你都在想这个？哇，你真是个深奥的思想家。对我而言，它只是一部电影罢了。"就像这样，虽然我的朋友感觉到我的情况有点异样，但他也只看得见这个表面症状。

As I got older, my manic, obsessive thoughts grew like wild fire. Movies were usually the spark. Once, while at work mowing the grass of a baseball field, my mind became obsessed with what I viewed as "subliminal messages" in the Disney movie, *Aladdin*. I was sure the makers of the movie unknowingly put hidden messages in the story line. It took several hours to mow that baseball field, but I was so engulfed in my thoughts, I didn't notice the time. When I finished mowing, I enthusiastically explained my thoughts to my work buddy. Instead of getting excited and enlightened as I had expected, he replied, "You thought about that this whole time? Man, you're a deep thinker. To me, it's just a movie." My friend recognized something wasn't normal, but he could only identify the surface symptom.

在儿童及青少年时期，一夜好眠往往能让那些躁狂的思绪缓和下来，促使躁郁症重新循环。当时我没有及早察觉躁狂症存在的情况下所遇到的危险是，我的躁狂强度与日俱增，越来越不想睡觉。睡眠不足是导致我在台湾严重发病的重要原因之一。除了这些强迫性的思绪或念头，躁狂症也把一些其他表面症状逐渐转变成我的个人特质。处于情绪巅峰状态的狂躁期让我外表上看起来非常热衷，动机旺盛，而且非常浪漫；像飞标钓鱼手一样富有创意，也跟他的钓钩一样锐利。认识我的人只觉得我是个"火药般"的人，完全没有料到我的精神即将爆炸。这其实是很典型的情况，许多像我一样发病的患者并不是人们以为的街头疯子，而是像高中毕业舞会的舞后，学生会主席，州辩论比赛的冠军，或是一个最佳运动员。

As a child and youth, a good night's sleep always slowed these manic thoughts down and reset the cycle. The danger I faced by not identifying my mania was, as time went on and the thoughts became more and more intense, I felt less and less like sleeping. Lack of sleep was one of the biggest factors preceding my extreme manic episode in Taiwan. Besides obsessive thinking, mania injected other surface symptoms into my personality. Being the "high" of the emotional cycle, mania made me appear extra enthusiastic, powerfully motivated, dynamically romantic, creative as a fly fisher, and sharp as his filed hook. Although everyone who knew me thought I was a "dynamite" person, no one expected my mental explosion. This is typical. Many people who suffer breakdowns similar to mine aren't the stereotypical "loony" on the street. They are the junior prom queens, the student body presidents, the state champion debaters, or the MVP athletes.

他们外在的表现都相当成功，直到体内未被察觉的躁狂症所累积的能量终于把他们推下现实的万丈悬崖。因此要察觉、确认躁郁症中躁狂的部分，就是要特别注意"极端"的情感表现，尤其当那些激动的情绪已经达到使人睡眠不足的时候。

提到睡眠，好，让我们现在把思索的速度放慢，慢慢来谈谈我的早期躁郁症的另一面极端，也就是"抑郁"的表面症状。

在我的记忆中，最初的抑郁经验也是在孩童时期，大约十或十一岁的时候。那时候我正要走到洗衣房时，心中突然有种强烈的一股气压袭来，或是重压我体内，一时忘记要去洗衣房拿什么。刚开始我以为那种感觉就是"担心"，于是我便停下来，在原地站了很久，想要回想起我到底在担心些什么。然而到最后，我还是没有想起来，因为我只是察觉表面上的症状，而完全没有察觉到真正的问题核心。

They are over‐achievers whose unidentified mania grows inside them until it shoves them off the cliff of reality. The way to identify bipolar mania is to be very weary of extremes in emotion, especially when those extremes lead to lack of sleep.

Sleep. Okay, now let's slow our thinking way down, talk slowly, and discuss my early surface symptoms on the other extreme of the bipolar scale：depression. The earliest I can remember depression was also during late childhood when I was ten or eleven years old. While walking toward the laundry room, I forgot what I was going to get because of an intense feeling or weight deep in my gut. I interpreted it to be worry. I stopped and stood there for a long time, trying to remember what I was worried about. It never came to me because I was only seeing the surface symptom and not identifying the real cause.

另一个使我误解抑郁症的表面症状是"罪恶感"，误把抑郁症当罪恶感，我开始相信我必须活得十全十美，才能避免这种罪恶感永远与我相伴。例如：我以前在学校读书时有一次经过一个垃圾桶，看到垃圾桶旁有一个被揉成球形的废纸，就像我常常投篮的结果——投了却投不进洞里。我对自己说："我应该把它捡起来丢进垃圾桶里。"却没有真的这样做。当我离开的时候，乌云般的罪恶感萦绕在我的脑中，像我们小时候把腐烂的鸡蛋丢到马厩墙壁上所产生的臭味一样无法散去。一个星期过后，那股罪恶感仍然挂在我心头。我觉得自己没有资格进入天国，因为就算我祷告请求宽恕，那种沮丧感仍然没有离开我。

Another surface symptom that my mind misinterpreted depression to be was guilt. Confusing depression for guilt, my mind started believing I had to live perfectly to avoid its constant companionship. For example, in school one day I walked by a trashcan. There was a wad of paper lying on the floor next to it, where, like many of my basketball shots, someone had missed. "I should pick that up," I thought to myself. As I walked away, a cloud of guilt swarmed around my mind like the smell of the rotten eggs we used to throw at the side of the barn. A week later, the stench of "guilt" still hung on me. I felt disqualified for heaven because even prayers begging for forgiveness didn't make the feeling go away.

为了让自己的抑郁显得很合理，我的脑袋开始发明一堆无谓的烦恼：我担心我的父母或兄弟姐妹会死亡、担心父亲会失业（虽然我爷爷是公司的大老板）、担心我的身体会突然变得畸形、担心将来长大后的出路……因为这未被察觉的抑郁症的存在，我的头脑几乎不间断地寻找着可以让我的担心或罪恶感能成立的一切理由，如果我找不到理由，便担心我为何不担心。很妙，是吧？

我的抑郁症第一次引起别人的注意，是在我读高中的时候。那是一个凉爽的秋夜，我去看一场高中美式橄榄球比赛，认识了一位美丽耀眼的红发女生。我们一起为我们支持的球队狂热地欢呼加油，在看台跳上跳下，并且放声大笑，完全听不见在我们后面想要坐着好好看比赛的父母们的怨言。

Searching for reasons, my mind started making up worries. I worried my parents or siblings were going to die. I worried my dad would lose his job (even though his dad owned the company). I worried about my body suddenly growing a deformity. I worried about not knowing what I would be when I grew up. With the unidentified depression always there, my brain constantly searched for things to worry or to feel guilty about. When I couldn't find a reason, I worried about not worrying. Fun, huh? The first time my bipolar surface symptoms drew comments from others happened when I was in high school. One cool, autumn evening I met a radiant redhead at a home football game. We had a blast cheering for our team, jumping up and down on the bleachers, and laughing loudly so we couldn't hear the upset comments of irritated parents behind us who preferred to watch the game while sitting.

一两天后，我再次见到那位红发女孩，我们在学校的走廊擦身而过。她静静地走来问我："怎么了？"这句话让我感到很迷惑，因为我一点都不觉得我有什么不对，为什么她会这么说呢？而当我又一次见到她时，她对我露出非常关心的表情，对我说："你在球赛的时候那么开心，但现在却看起来很难过！你到底怎么了？"

如果我能回到过去、回答她的问题的话，我会告诉她，在球赛那天晚上我正处于躁狂情绪飙高的状态中，但两天后的我则是处在轻度的抑郁状态，所以看起来很难过的样子。但当时我完全不知道是怎么回事，只是觉得那个女生很奇怪；而她呢，大概会认为我精神有问题吧！如果她是这样想的话，她其实是正确的，而我自己则要到几年之后才察觉这个问题。

The next time I saw her was a couple of days later when we passed each other in the hall at school. She quietly walked up to me and asked, "What's wrong?" Her words confused me. I didn't feel like anything was wrong. Why did she say that? The next time I saw her, she got a deep, concerned look on her face and said, "You were so happy at the football game and now you're so sad! What's wrong?" If I could go back and answer her question now, I would tell her that I had been on a manic high the night of the football game. And that now I was in my usual, mild depression mode. That's why I looked sad. But I didn't know, I just thought she was weird. She probably thought I was mental. If that's what she thought, she was right. But I wouldn't identify it for a few more years.

从那时起，我开始注意到别人常常会对我说我看起来很累，有时他们会问我："你还好吗？"我学会用不客气的口气很快地回答："不用管我，我只是累了。"而因为我这千篇一律、令人恼火的回答，后来就没有人想继续关心我的状况。我总是想办法终结话题，避免谈到我哪里不舒服，或是允许别人知道或帮助我察觉我的抑郁——后来我发觉，如果一位平常性情温和且有耐心的人突然变得易怒，也可能是躁郁症引起的症状。说到逃避痛苦，躁郁症的另外一项表面症状，是在我还是青少年时就开始遭受到的，我自己称之为"可怕思想（scary thoughts）"，虽然后来听到医生说正确的说法应该是"intrusive thoughts（侵入式思想）"，但我觉得自己的说法形容得更贴近真实。

From that time on, I began to notice people constantly commenting that I looked tired. They sometimes asked me if I was okay. I learned just to snap back, "Don't worry about me. I'm just tired." With this annoyed, standard answer no one ever pressed the issue further, and I always managed to end the conversation without digging where it hurt or allowing others to see or help identify my depression. Come to find out, irritability from a person who is usually agreeable and patient can also be a surface symptom of bipolar disorder. Speaking of avoiding pain, another surface symptom of bipolar disorder, something which started pecking at me in my late youth was what I termed: "scary thoughts." I later learned the medical term to be "intrusive thoughts." I think my term is a more accurate description.

许多精神科医生以及社工相信，"可怕思想"实际上是一种心理的分裂：他们说头脑就像是一个去农场玩却被公鸡攻击的小孩子。事后，他如果没有撒野一番他是绝对不会再去那个农场的。"抑郁"就是那只凶狠的公鸡；与其一次又一次遭遇到抑郁的折磨，头脑学会用比撒野更有力量、更有控制力的想法来控制。

但我的母亲不这样想，她坚信是魔鬼把那些可怕的思想放进我的脑袋里；至于我，我不知道我的情况属于哪一种，或者两种说法都有一些吧。我确知的是，魔鬼思想已开始在我青少年时期时时恐吓我。

到底"可怕思想"是什么呢？我觉得最好且最明白的解释就是，我的脑袋里总是卡着一个问题："在任何的情况下，我所能做到或说出最糟糕的东西是什么？"

Many psychiatrists and social workers believe that scary thoughts are actually mental distractions. They say the brain is like a child who is attacked and hurt by the barnyard rooster. The child will never go to the barnyard again without throwing a fit. Depression is the barnyard rooster. Rather than deal with its accompanying pain and anguish over and over again, the brain learns to "throw fits" in order to occupy itself with more powerful and controlling thoughts. My mother thinks differently. She believes scary thoughts are put in my head by the devil. I don't know which is the case or if it's a combination of both. I do know that demonic thoughts started haunting me during my late teenage years. So what were they? I guess the best way to describe them would be to say that somehow my brain got stuck on the question, "What is the worst possible thing I could do or say in any given situation?"

这个可怕问题的答案不定时地在我的脑海里飕飕地飞来飞去，就像某个在山上露营的夜晚，当我调皮的朋友偷偷把一些0.22的小子弹丢进营火里一样。子弹受热、开始往四处弹射时，我们赶紧找石头及树木掩护自己。容我举一些例子：当我站在五百英尺高的山峰上俯瞰美丽的包威尔湖（Lake Powell）时，咻！一个自杀念头在我耳边悄声说："往下跳！"当我在上课，数学老师经过我的桌子时，飕！一个暴力而凶狠的声音对我说："痛打他一拳！"当我坐在教堂里，正聆听一篇关于如何避免说出亵渎言语的演讲时，唰！有个奇异的声音催促我："大声喊脏话！"而当我参加宴会，坐在父亲的头号客户的隔壁用餐时，嘶！一个粗鲁无礼的思想强迫我："在客人的食物上吐口水！"——其实这些只是几个很温和的例子，我想我不需要写出更黑暗、更可怕或更极端的例子。

Answers to this horrifying question randomly whizzed through my head like the time my buddy foolishly snuck a handful of 0.22 bullets into our campfire. We all jumped for cover behind rocks and trees when the bullets heated up and started shooting through the air. Zing; a suicidal thought whispered, "Jump!" when I stood on top of a 500-foot cliff overlooking Lake Powell. Zang; a violent thought growled, "Punch him where it hurts!" when my math teacher walked past my desk. Zoom; a totally bizarre thought urged, "Yell cuss words!" when I sat in church listening to a talk on avoiding profanity. Kazowie; a rude thought tempted, "Spit in his food!" when I sat next to one of my dad's top clients at a formal banquet. These are examples of *mild* scary thoughts. I don't think it is necessary to share the darker, more extreme ones.

当这些骇人的思想像子弹一样射进我的脑海时，我不知道它们从哪儿来，更不晓得该如何应对和处理，我不敢跟任何人谈起这些想法，因为我害怕被别人视为疯子或恶魔。抗拒且不打算寻求帮助的我，宁可把这些恐怖思想藏进脑海深处，并因此时常感到罪恶与烦恼。我从来没有按照那些可怕的思想去行动，只是假装它们不存在。

另一个逐渐发展的失调状况所表现的表面症状——上瘾。许多患有躁郁症的人为了逃避抑郁之苦，会滥用毒品或酒，我知道服用那些不好，所以我开始依赖另一个"合法"的东西，那东西就像毒品及酒精一样，对我的身心都有效，能让我早上顺利起床、晚上安稳睡着，在运动时更能提振我的精神，并且在比赛中帮助我进步更多。简单地说，它在我一切的活动中帮助提升我的情绪。

When the scary thoughts started shooting at me, I had no idea where they came from or what to do about them. I didn't dare talk about them with anyone because I feared people would think I was crazy or evil. Rather than seek help, I repressed them away deep in my mind, all the while feeling guilty and worried. I never acted on the thoughts; I just pretended they didn't exist.

Another surface symptom of my developing disorder was an addiction. Many people who have bipolar illness abuse drugs or alcohol to escape the agony of depression. I knew these were wrong. I became dependant on another "legal" substance. This substance had as much power on my mind and body as drugs or alcohol. It got me going in the morning and settled me down at night. It pumped me up when I exercised and helped improve my athletic performance. It enhanced my emotions in all my activities.

在我青少年的时候，我就照着 Journey 乐团的歌所说的"open arms"（敞开双臂）邀请这东西——也就是音乐——进入我的心中。我不是说音乐不好，只是音乐的节奏、和声，以及音量，都对我有相当大的影响力。对我而言，它跟咖啡因有相同的效果。在我青少年时期，一天到晚听音乐，能让我大部分时间的心情得以从沉重的不安或罪恶感中"飘浮"，协助我释放忧虑。

写到这里，我想重复一件非常重要的事：当你读到我这些早期躁郁症的表面症状，你很可能对自己说："我感觉我的生活中也有这些全部症状。我的血液里是否也有躁郁症在暗自沸腾，随时准备要爆炸？"不用担心，也别急着跑医院检查，不是每个脑中常听到音乐，或因想事情而失眠的人都患了躁郁症。

During my teenage years it became an addiction that I invited in with, as Journey sang, "open arms." The substance was music. I'm not saying the music was bad. I'm saying the beat, the harmonies, and the volume affected me profoundly. It literally had the same effect as caffeine. Constantly listening to music enabled me to float above guilt and blast out worried thoughts most of the time during my teenage years. I want to reiterate something very important here. As you read my early mania and depression surface symptoms, you probably thought to yourself, "I have felt all of these at different times in my life. Do I have bipolar disorder boiling in my blood, just waiting to explode?" Don't worry. Don't run down and check yourself into a hospital. Not everyone who gets songs stuck in their head, or who loses sleep because something is on their mind has bipolar disorder.

大部分脑中有不愉快或可怕思想的人，总为一些傻事杞人忧天，或因小错而愧疚不已的人，以及会毫无理由地发脾气，或偶尔感到被沮丧重重压住肠胃的人，其实并没有罹患躁郁症。请记住，每一个人都多少会经历一些轻微的症状，躁郁症是一种因为脑内化学物质不平衡而造成生理上的极端行为表现。借着过简单而基本的健康生活——规律运动、适当睡眠、良好的饮食习惯加上控制压力，大部分的人不会被严重的躁狂症，或被深深且持续的抑郁症缠上。青少年时期以来，随着成长，我的躁狂跟抑郁越来越严重。只能看到表面症状的我，没有发现或了解真正的原因，一点都没有想过这些症状可能是头脑里面有精神病在扩大的征兆。

Most people who have unpleasant or scary thoughts, who worry about silly things, who feel big guilt for small mistakes, who get irritated for unseen reasons, or who sometimes feel the wrenching weight of depression pushing down on their gut do not have bipolar disorder. Remember, *everyone* experiences mild symptoms. Bipolar disorder is a chemical imbalance in the brain that physically forces untreated symptoms to the extreme. By living a simple, basic, healthy lifestyle of regular exercise, proper sleep, good diet, and controlled stress, most people do not fall victim to extreme mania or deep, lasting depression. As I grew into the later teenage years, my mania and depression became more and more extreme. Only seeing the surface symptoms, I didn't recognize or understand the true source. I never considered the possibility that the surface symptoms could be indicators of a growing mental illness.

其他人——像我的父母、高中时那位红头发的可爱女生、帮我一起除草的朋友——都注意到我的状况；他们不知道那是什么情形，但他们知道是不正常的。假如我能和他们真诚地沟通，听听他们的意见，还有多注意他们对我的观察的话，必然能帮助我提早几年在我被吹离这个星球之前，认清我的疾病。大多数没有接受治疗的躁郁症患者，其"躁狂—抑郁"的无尽循环，会在从青少年转为成人的过程中不断加重。就像我一样，它不是一眨眼就会变得不可收拾，而是要经过好几年，像从外太空飞来地球的微小物体一样，它的亮度增加得非常慢，所以没有人注意到它。当我在台湾参加志愿服务时我那不明原因的疯狂逐渐蓄势爆发时，没有人意料到它的来临。

Others, like my parents, the cute redhead at high school, and my lawn-mowing buddy did notice. They didn't know what it was, but they knew it wasn't normal. Honest communication, simply listening to them, and paying attention to their observations could have helped me identify the illness years before it blew me off the planet. For most people with untreated bipolar disorder, the manic-depressive cycle intensifies through youth and into early adulthood as mine did. It doesn't happen all at once. Over many years, it grows like the view of a tiny object in space, hurtling toward earth. The flaming light grows brighter and bigger so slowly that no one pays attention to it. When my UFO (Unidentified Freak Out) crashed down during my volunteer work in Taiwan, no one knew it was coming.

　　我那次躁狂的"爆发"有着出乎意料的力量，让许多人都被波及，在那之后，察觉我的疾病只是时间的问题。很显然地，早点察觉这种疾病的存在，是可以预防它走向极端与爆发的关键；然而不管心理疾病在哪个阶段被察觉，几乎都是可以治疗的。好比你跟朋友们划船时有人落水，即使他沉到水里，甚至有一两分钟停止呼吸，你还是可以用CPR（人工呼吸）来救他一样。当年发病的我，可以说是被心理疾病的急流卷进漩涡的最深处，但是我终究能够再次浮上水面，呼吸到带来美好生命的空气。为了到达逃离心理疾病急流的第一块踏脚石"察觉"，首先我必须回顾过往的表面症状，从中辨认出心理疾病的真面目，而且即使是到了这一步，之后也还有很长的路要走。

　　The manic explosion hit with such unexpected power, it forced many people to get involved. After that, identifying the cause was only a matter of time. Obviously, identifying the illness early is the key to preventing extreme episodes. However, no matter what stage mental illness is identified in, it is almost always treatable. If you're river rafting with a group and someone falls overboard, even if he stays under so long that he stops breathing for a minute or two, you can still revive him with CPR. I can say the mental illness rapids sucked me into the cyclone about as deep as it gets. And yet, I was still able to come back up and find the breath of life again. In order to reach "Identify," the first stepping-stone out of the mental illness rapids, I first needed to see past the surface symptoms and recognize mental illness for what it was. Even then, I still had a long way to go.

当我站在"察觉"的踏脚石上，那仿佛达到国际水域分级第六级（最危险）的心理疾病急流不断在我的四周咆哮，让我听不见"你已身陷心理疾病"的微小提醒。换句话说，"知道"我得了躁郁症（被心理疾病激流围困），跟愿意"承认"它的确存在于我的生命的事实，完全是两码事。"承认"是帮助我逃离心理疾病症急流的第二块必要的踏脚石。

While standing on "Identify," the roaring reality of the grade VI manic-depressive rapids all around me made me deaf to the voice that told me I was mentally ill. In other words, knowing I had bipolar disorder and authorizing it into my life were two different things. Reaching this "authorization" turned out to be the second necessary step to get me out of the mental illness rapids.

第三章　步骤二：承认你的疾病

心理疾病的确改变了我

我现在是个更好的人

想象你某天早上在一片又干又热的沙漠中醒来，在沙地中矗立、长得像"哥布林"（一种西方传说中的精怪生物：goblin）的红色与褐色砂岩巨石似乎是你唯一的"同伴"。突然，一位穿白色医生袍的人从一尊看起来又哭又笑的怪异哥布林巨石后面出现，走过来给你一块大石头，他深深盯着你的眼睛说："你必须带着这个。"然后二话不说地从巨石的后面消失。你很快会发现他给你的石头非常重，当你在沙漠中跋涉好几公里，试着找寻出口时，你还得用极大的力气把那块石头扛在身上。

Chapter 3
Step Two：Authorize Your Illness into Your Life

Yes, mental illness changed me

Now I'm a better person

Imagine yourself waking up one morning in the middle of a hot, dry desert. Towering red and brown, goblin-like sandstone sculptures shooting out of the sandy floor seem to be the only company around. Suddenly, a man dressed in white hospital scrubs walks out from behind a particularly creepy sand goblin – one that looks like it is laughing and crying at the same time – and hands you a large stone. Looking deeply into your eyes he says, "You must carry this with you." Without another word he disappears back into the sandstone maze. You quickly realize the rock he gave you is quite heavy. Still, with great effort, you carry it along as you drift for miles in the sand trying to find a way out.

日正当午，炽热的太阳没多久就逼走所有巨石底下的凉荫。低头看看，你见到你自己的脚印，发现自己只是在原地打转。沮丧的你开始诅咒起高热的太阳和沙子，还有你一直扛在身上的笨石头。在仅存的一点阴影里，你坐下来认真思考，终于你想到："或许我该好好看看这块石头，也许那人是想帮我一把！"这是你首次仔细端详你抱那么久的沉重石头，令你惊讶的是石头上原来刻着非常翔实的地图。你研究地图，看到离你不远处有个小径的入口，那小径最后会引你到一个有人烟的湖边。旅途虽长，但沿路有食物及饮水。你对于有希望能得救的第一个反应是满怀喜悦感激，但再深入研究地图后，你又发现抵达湖边之前有许多岔路，误入歧途的结果将会陷入绝地或险境。你理解此情况后，再度感到不安。

It isn't long before the burning sun dries up the shade of the sandstone goblins around you. Looking down, you discover your own footprints and realize you are wandering in circles. In frustration you curse the heat, the sand, and the stupid rock you are carrying. You sit down in one of the last slivers of shade to really think. Finally, it occurs to you. Maybe I should look at the rock. Perhaps the man was trying to help! For the first time, you take a good look at the heavy stone you have been packing around for so long. To your surprise, you identify a very detailed map carved into the rock. You study the map and discover a trailhead not far from where you are. The trail leads to a lake where there is civilization. The journey will take a long time but there is food and water along the way. Your first reaction is joy and gratitude at the opportunity to be saved. However, as you study the map further, you see that before the trail gets to the lake, there are several forks to be navigated. With anguish, you see that a wrong choice could lead you to perilous and hazardous areas.

你自知无法记住到那座湖边的完整路线，因此必须继续带着大石头前进。当你开始按照地图指示走上小径时，心里不禁怀疑："那位穿着医生袍的人究竟是敌是友？"

而当你来到小路的第一个岔路时，你看到有另外一个人在那儿，她也带着一块刻有地图的重石头；她的石头有不同的形状和颜色，但看来和你的石头等重，甚至比你的更重。那位女子对你露出微笑，然后拿起她的石头继续她的行程；在你持续前进的路上，你看到更多也带着重石头的人。有些人微笑着，但多数的人喃喃抱怨；在你漫长的旅途中，你也曾遇上残忍的野兽及充满考验的地形，每个障碍都好像是为了毁灭你而设。然而当你每次跟它们搏斗时，你都能发掘足够的力量来克服挑战。最后，你终于明白了——让你变得强壮、足以克服一切挑战，而安全到达天堂般的湖边的原因，就是因为你一直扛着那块大石头。

Knowing you won't be able to remember all of the directions that lead you safely to the lake, you realize you'll still have to carry the heavy rock with you. As you start down the trail you wonder, "Was the man in scrubs my friend or my foe?" As you come to the first fork in the trail, you see another person there. She also has a heavy rock with a map on it. Her rock is a different shape and a different color, but it looks just as heavy or maybe even heavier than yours. She smiles at you, picks up her rock and continues on her way. Continuing on, you see many other people, each carrying his or her own rock. Some smile. Many murmur. On the trail of your long journey, you also encounter bloodthirsty beasts and testing terrain. Each obstacle seems to be set on your destruction. Every time you wrestle with them, however, you find the strength necessary to come out conqueror. Finally, you figure it all out. Carrying your rock is what makes you strong enough to overcome all the challenges and safely reach the heavenly lake.

　　我分享这个"石头寓言"，以利描述我"承认心理疾病在我生命中确实存在"的这个困难决定。发现石头上的地图，就好像是察觉我的生活里存在着必须面对的疾病，一旦察觉之后，就不可能把它丢下不管。那时我完全不晓得这个笨重包袱怎么可能帮助我变得更坚强，所以我面对的新问题是："我要用什么态度来带着这个新的重担生活下去？"但愿我能告诉你我是用微笑的双眼和轻松的口哨来面对它，可惜我不是，我反而凶神恶煞地骂那些试图帮助我的人。第一个倒霉的人（就是我中止在中国台湾的志愿服务，被送回美国老家附近的医院之后）就是我的精神科医生。

I share this "parable of the rock" to help describe the difficult decision to allow, or authorize, mental illness into my life. Discovering the map on the rock was like identifying the illness. Once identified, I couldn't just leave the disorder behind. At that point, I couldn't see how such "heavy baggage" could ever make me stronger. So, the new question I faced was, "What attitude will I choose as I carry this hefty burden with me?" I wish I could say I set out with smiling eyes and whistling lips…but I can't. Instead, with a snarl in my voice and a scowl on my face, I lashed out at those who tried to help me. First in line (after I was sent home from my volunteer service in Chinese Taiwan to the psychiatric ward of a hospital near my home) was my psychiatrist.

　　大约住院一个礼拜后的某一天，在我们每天例行的散步谈话中，我向医生吐露我从来没有告诉过任何人的事。我提到了我的"可怕思想"，特别是读高中时催促我朝经过我座位的老师身体最敏感的部位痛打下去的可怕念头。几天之后，医生提到医疗委员会针对我的可怕思想讨论了一些东西。"你跟其他人说了？"我像个信号弹般，情绪失控地对医生尖叫起来。"是的，我以为你知道，我们会有一个由医疗专家组成的医疗委员会，针对我们散步时所谈到的发现来讨论，希望能给你最好的药物和治疗。"医生如此辩解。"我以为我们是朋友！"我反击他的说辞："你一点也不在乎我，你只不过是在履行你的工作，当我走了之后你就会忘记我！"

　　"我是你的朋友。"他说着，但带着一丝防卫的眼神："我想给你最好的治疗。"

　　After a week or so, on one of our daily walk – and – talks, I confided to him something I had never told anyone. I told him about my scary thoughts, specifically the urge I had in high school to punch my teacher in the sensitive spot when he walked past my desk. A few days later he mentioned something about the medical committee discussing my scary thoughts. "You told other people?" I screeched, like a signal flare calling all my emotions to the front line. "Yes, I thought you knew there is a whole committee of medical professionals who discuss the findings from our walks and try to come up with the best medication and treatment for you." he defended.

　　"I thought we were friends!" I fired back. "You don't care about me, you're just doing your job and when I am gone you will forget me."

　　"I am your friend," he said with a shielded look in his eye. "I want what is best for you."

"朋友绝不会随便对别人说出他朋友的秘密！"我如此回答，同时拼命试着不让泪水夺眶而出。从那次的"误解战争"之后，我完全不再信赖他的专业知识及经验，相反地，我开始讨厌他。有整整一个月的时间，我责怪他不允许我出院以继续我的志愿服务。从那时起，我总带着"否认"的狙击枪，迅速地击落来自医生所尝试的任何协助或建议，我开始像一位……嗯，就说是"疯子"吧，极力保护着我心中真正的情感。

我当时想要保护深锁在我发狂脑袋中的秘密，是那引发我精神崩溃的幻想狂热。当时我不愿意承认医生所诊断出来的结果（罹患躁郁症），反而相信自己才是唯一真正了解我在台湾发生了什么事的人——我的头脑确信自己遭遇到超自然的非肉体经验，而不是精神崩溃。

"Friends don't go around blabbing secrets about their friends to others." I said, fighting desperately to hold back the mounting tears. After that battle of misunderstanding, I completely stopped trusting his knowledge and experience. Rather, I started to despise him. For a whole month I blamed him for not approving me to leave the hospital and continue my volunteer service. From then on, with the sniper rifle of denial, I immediately shot down any assistance or counsel the doctor tried to approach me with. I started guarding my true feelings and emotions like a…well…a maniac. The thing I was protecting, locked deep inside my ill mind, was a secret belief in the fanatic obsessions that had sparked my extreme manic breakdown. Not authorizing the illness the doctor had identified allowed my mind to believe I was the only one who really understood the episode in Taiwan. My mind became convinced that what really happened was a supernatural, out-of-body experience, not a mental breakdown.

　　有好几个星期，我假装听进医生说的每一句话，而且夸张地说他所建议的康复对我多么有效，我唯一渴望的就是让他允许我出院。我不知道是否我骗过了他还是我欺骗了自己，住院一个月之后，医生终于勉强同意我出院，并说："我会让你离开，但恐怕你会很快地被送回这儿。"此后，我就重新被派到蒙大拿州继续我的志愿服务，在我停药后没多久，我的病果真再度严重发作。这次我的父母很仁慈地决定带我回家，不再把我送到精神病院。他们完全不知道（也许他们知道，但仍带我回家）这样做会让他们成为我唇枪舌剑无辜的牺牲者。我回家后几天，母亲虽然早已料到，但她还是故意问了我："安迪，你今晚吃药了吗？"

For weeks, I pretended to listen to everything the doctor said and I exaggerated my improvement from his recommended therapy. All I really wanted was his permission to leave. I don't know if I fooled him, or if I was just fooling myself, but a month later my doctor reluctantly signed my release with the words, "I'll let you go, but I'm afraid you'll end up right back here." I was reassigned to Montana to continue my service. It wasn't long before I quit taking my medication and the second extreme manic episode followed. This time, my mother and father lovingly decided to bring me home instead of check me into another hospital. They didn't realize (or maybe they did and brought me home anyway) this put them next in line for my firing squad. "Andy, have you taken your medication tonight?" My mother asked a few days later, knowing full well I had not.

"那不是药！它只是给我的头脑的化学制品！"我朝她吼着："我不需要吃药，我只是需要化学制品！"我只选择听我想听的话，好让我的控制欲得到不切实际的满足，同时让我觉得需要帮助的人并不是我而是她。指出别人的弱点跟错误很快地成为我的恶习，使我远离当时迫切需要的援助与"化学制品"，结果我后来再受多次精神崩溃之苦的时候，倍感孤单无助。否认躁郁症的存在所造成的病情延误和人际关系破裂，只是问题的一半而已；白天的严重抑郁远比晚上的躁狂发作更糟，那感觉好像是沉重的水泥车天天压着我的身与心。新的精神科医生常关切我抑郁的程度有多严重，还询问我需不需要吃抗抑郁的药物，然而我并不愿意接受、也不愿承认使我每天早晨下床难如登天的抑郁症。

"It's not medication! It's just chemicals for my brain." I yelled at her. "I don't need medication. I just need chemicals." Forcing my mother to say the words I wanted her to say gave me a false sense of control. It made me feel like she was the one who needed help, not me. Pointing out the weaknesses and faults of others soon became an ugly habit that dragged me away from the help and the "chemicals" I so desperately needed. Consequently, I felt alone as I suffered many more manic breakdowns. Untreated mania and damaged relationships were only half of the problem resulting from not authorizing the illness into my life. Even worse than the nighttime manic breakdowns, heavy depression weighed down my mind and body every day like a truckload of wet cement. My new psychiatrist often asked what my depression level was and if I needed antidepressant medication. But I wouldn't admit or even acknowledge that it was depression that made getting out of bed each morning so tough.

　　所以我说谎欺骗医生，假装我的生活跟沐浴着春光飞来飞去的蝴蝶一样无忧无虑。

　　事实上，缺少抗抑郁药物的我的心理状态，就像是一只在寒冬的黑暗山洞里冬眠的蝙蝠一样晦暗死寂。我大部分的早上及下午是躺在床上或沙发上，一个小时接着一个小时，一天又一天。虽然我的行为几乎和几年前的母亲一模一样，但我那时候还不愿意承认自己跟她相同。我不愿承认那种让母亲看来那么脆弱的"病情"进入我自己的生命。很快地，睡觉变成我唯一的逃避方式，每次起床，我感觉自己的身体像一辆在寒冷中试着发动的柴油大卡车那样难以运转，所以我每天都赖床直到下午很晚的时候（没错，是下午），把午餐当成早餐吃，然后赶到我父亲的建筑工地上夜班。

So I lied and I pretended my life was as bright and shiny as a butterfly fluttering around in springtime sunbeams. In actuality, with no antidepressant medication my emotions were more like a bat in a dark cave hibernating through a bitter winter. I spent most of my mornings and afternoons lying in bed or on the couch, day after day, hour after hour. Although my actions were almost identical to what my mother's had been just a few years earlier, I refused to admit I was like her. I would not authorize the "condition" that made my mother seem so weak into my own life. Soon, sleep became the only escape I could find. Waking up, my body felt like an 18-wheel diesel rig trying to get started in freezing temperatures. I dragged out of bed late each afternoon (that's not a typo), ate lunch for breakfast, and then rushed to work doing a night watch job at my dad's construction site.

　　一般建筑员工下班的时间是下午三点半。我照理应该在他们离开的时候就到达工地。但是有太多次，我都因为睡觉爬不起来以至于在下午四点半或五点之后才到。往往我会开车到充满灰尘的地方，确认周围都没有人后，把车椅放平再睡上一两个小时。

　　许多重度的抑郁症患者会用非法毒品，或是喝酒来逃避他们的病情。我知道不该那样做，所以从未把它们当作选择，但是我嗜睡的习惯开始对我的身体产生了与滥用毒品类似的影响：我睡得越多，起床时的抑郁就越严重，而我的抑郁越严重，我就越想要睡，我称这个现象为"杀手循环"。

　　让我试着描述从过长的睡眠中醒来时，那种极端抑郁的感觉：我全身紧张又激动，起床做些什么事的动力和对世界的兴趣都是难以忍受的巨大负担，所以我干脆把它们当成发黑的香蕉皮或发酸的牛奶盒一样扔得老远。

Quitting time for the construction workers was 3：30 PM. I was supposed to be there when they left. Many times, I arrived after 4：30 or 5：00 because I couldn't get out of bed in time. Often, I'd pull into the dusty site, look around to make sure no one was there, then lay back the seat in my car and fall asleep for another hour or two. Many severely depressed people use illegal drugs or alcohol as an escape. I knew these were wrong and never considered them an option. However, my addiction to sleep started having the same effect on my body as abused drugs. The more I slept, the more severe the depression was when I woke up. The more severe the depression, the more I longed for sleep. I came to call this "the killer cycle." Let me try to describe the feeling of extreme depression after waking up from too much sleep. My whole body was tense and agitated. My motivation to get up and do things and my interest in the world felt like cumbersome loads that were too heavy to carry; so I tossed them out like black banana peels and sour milk cartons.

　　我的手脚很想运动，但我的头却深感筋疲力尽而难以动弹，我的肚子因为睡得太多而错过用餐，总是饿得大声咕噜叫，但是食物的样子让我作呕，我几乎没有食欲。

　　麦当劳的广告、NBA 篮球赛（是在介绍球员的时候，而非我支持的球队输了）、高中田径赛，以及听到哭丧的乡村音乐都会让我哭出来。有时候我忘记自己有没有笑过，或是否曾有过其他感受；有时甚至接下来的五分钟，也如未来一般遥远；极端的抑郁持续恐吓着我，当听到新闻报道加州帮派要求想加入的人必须先杀人的时候，我就害怕被杀。虽然我在离他们好远的犹他州，一点危险性都没有，但我的脑海却一直萦绕着这件事，真的相信一不小心就会被杀了。

　　My hands and legs tingled and itched for exercise, but my head was too exhausted and heavy to move. My stomach screamed of starvation from meals missed while sleeping, but food looked revolting and I rarely had an appetite. I bawled over McDonalds' commercials, NBA basketball games (not when my team lost, but when they introduced the players), high school track meets, and listening to sappy country music. At times I forgot I had ever laughed or that I had ever felt different. Sometimes, the next five minutes were as far into the future as I could see. Extreme worry haunted my mind continually. I remember fearing death following a news report about California gangsters receiving initiation on the streets. Even though I was in rural Utah and the threat to me was non-existent, my mind mulled over the story so much, I really feared that one wrong move could get me killed.

就像射到石头上的子弹又反弹回来，我之前向母亲射出的话也被反弹回我的耳朵。人们往往告诉我"只要别想那么多就好了，只要多微笑，只要早一点睡觉就能早一点起床。"我发觉自己无法照他们的话做。每天抑郁像大公牛一般把我撞倒的时候，我唯一逃避的方法就是赶快睡觉。当早上需要前往某处的时候，我便牺牲洗澡、刷牙、刮胡子的时间，来换取更长的睡眠时间。礼拜天补习在上午十一点半才开始，但我认为这时间很早；穿着未烫的衣服、没梳好头发的我，通常在十二点二十五分——刚好在老师讲完课的同时——才到学校；有许多个礼拜天我甚至起不了床，根本没有到补习班去。

秋季上大学时也是一样的情况：我选的是近午以及下午的课，却仍常迟到或根本就跷课不去。过度的睡眠也使我的健康受到不良影响，因为我把睡觉看得比吃饭更重要。

Like a ricocheting echo to the words I shot at my mother a few years earlier, people often told me, "Just don't think so much. Just smile more. Just go to bed earlier; then you can get up sooner." I found it impossible to do so. Each day when depression knocked me down with the power of a hungry bull, hitting the hay was the only escape I could find. When I had to be somewhere, I sacrificed showering and grooming so I could sleep a little longer. On Sundays, the early morning study school started at 11：30. I usually showed up, all scruffy, with wrinkled clothes, at 12：25, just as the teacher was finishing the last lesson. Many Sundays, I never made it to study school at all. Same story when school began in the fall. I signed up for late morning and even afternoon classes, but often arrived tardy or missed them altogether. Oversleeping also negatively affected my health by taking precedence over eating.

在那段难受的时期，我参加了一个跑步比赛，在那儿可以做一次健康分析。检查的结果是，我160磅的体重里面，有156磅瘦肉，3.5磅脂肪——我的身体只有2.2%是肥肉而已！报告还说到，按照我的年龄与性别来看，我的这种身体情况是有风险的。对，没错，但我还是选择睡觉而不吃东西。善良而想帮我快乐起来的好友们常带我去那些我曾喜欢去的地方，可惜这些旅游往往达不到效果。比如有一次，钓鱼的伙伴带我去河钓，以为这样会使我开心起来，我们分开两三个小时他回到我身边，以为会见到我正放松而愉快地钓鱼，但却找到在太阳下晒伤的我沉睡在一座桥上。还有一次，合唱课里的一位女生以为买票带我去看我很喜欢的乐团的演唱会让我微笑起来。

At a road race during that difficult time, I had a fitness analyses done. The results said, of my 160 pounds of weight, I was 97.8%, or 156.5 pounds lean, and 3.5 pounds fat. My body only had 2.2% fat! The report went on to state that my fitness rating as a percentile of the population in my age and gender group, was risky. Yeah, I'd say so. Yet, I continued choosing sleep over meals. Thoughtful friends tried to cheer me up by taking me on outings to places I used to love. Sadly, these outings often ended in disaster – like the time my fishing buddy tried to cheer me up by taking me to our favorite river. After we split up for a couple of hours, instead of finding me relaxed and happily fly fishing, he stumbled upon me baking in the sun, sound asleep on a bridge. Another time a girl in my choir class thought she could put a smile on my face by buying tickets and taking me to one of my favorite music group's concerts.

　　我可以想象当时她不得不把闪光灯的影子当成舞伴，而我则一个人坐在看台椅子上，把头埋在手里时，她的内心有多么失望。每当抑郁症发作时，我就没有心情跳舞、钓鱼、唱歌，或从事任何其他活动——除了睡觉以外。抑郁一直困扰着我，不论去哪里或做什么它都赖在我身上。大部分时间它的力量强大到让我无法踏出家门。假如你是躁郁症病患的照顾者或家人，你应该就遇到过与上述因不愿面对患病事实的态度带来的否认、恨意和不愿意参加活动（抽离原本生活）等等类似情形。遇上这些情形时，你怎么帮助你所爱的人接受现实呢？答案就是：耐心。

I can only imagine how disappointed she was when she had to settle for her strobe-light shadow as a dancing partner while I sat alone in the bleachers with my head in my hands. When deep depression struck, I didn't feel like dancing, fishing, singing, or anything except sleeping. When it latched on, it stuck with me no matter where I went or what I did. Most of the time, it was too powerful to even leave the house. If you are a caregiver for, or a family member of, a person with bipolar disorder, chances are you have encountered similar situations of denial, resentment, and withdrawal resulting from unwillingness to authorize the illness into his or her life. So how can you help your loved one to accept reality? The answer is patience.

心理疾病就像一座可以烧掉固执、骄傲这类负面特质的火炉，有个方法可以让你增加耐力，那就是试着去了解：叫一个有心理疾病的人相信你，胜过相信他自己，对他来说是多么困难的一件事！假如你的心情正高兴、快乐得不得了的时候（虽然是凌晨三点），而有人却说你是在发躁狂症状，说你有病，你会怎样呢？如果你感到悲哀沉闷，了无生趣，你的父母或其他亲友却告诉你其实一切没那么糟糕，你只是头脑里有不正常的化学反应在作祟而已，你有办法相信吗？很难想象，对不对？

The fiery furnacemental illness is will eventually burn away the impurities of stubbornness and pride. One way to build your endurance is to come to understand how difficult it is for the mentally ill person to believe you more than believing her own mind. Think about that for a minute. What would it take for you to trust another person more than your own mind? If you were feeling great, high and at the top of your game (even though it was 3：00 in the morning), and someone said you were manic and ill, how would you take it? If you felt so down and blue, like all hope was lost and your life was in shambles, would you believe it if your parents or friends assured you everything was fine and you were simply suffering from imbalanced chemicals in your brain? It's hard to imagine, isn't it?

这就是为什么可能要单方面付出好几年的耐性、宽容，还有不断坚持的爱心，才能得到病患的信任，好让他不保留地接受你的意见。我父母及家人帮我的成功方法，就是一直把我当成一个健全、善良的人。他们知道我对他们发脾气或不愿意参加活动，是因为我的疾病，而不是我的本意。他们从未逼我张嘴吃药，也从未大声对我不愿听见的耳朵喊出批评的话，而且从未把现实硬塞进我困惑的脑海里。这样，我才渐渐相信他们对我的爱，进而信任他们所提供的协助。不过，当我建议耐心是帮助你所爱的人治疗躁郁症的方式的同时，我也明白就算是最有耐心的照顾者也是有限度的。有时候，心理疾病的患者非常极端的行为，会超越照顾者能承受的范围，这时把他们所爱的患者送到精神病院，或离婚，或将他们与父母分开，都是无可避免的结果。

This is why it may take years of patience, forgiveness, and unyielding love on your part before the mentally ill person will gain the amount of trust necessary to blindly follow your counsel. The way my parents and family did it was to always believe and treat me like I was a good and kind person. They knew the aggression and withdrawal were results of my illness and not the real me. They never forced pills through my clenched teeth. They never cranked criticism through my pinched ears. And they never rammed reality into my bewildered brain. As a result, I came to believe in their love and to trust their offerings of help. Now, when I recommend patience as the solution to helping a loved one accept and authorize his or her illness, I realize even the most patient caregivers have limits. Sometimes people with mental illness abuse others in such extremes that hospitalization, divorce, or even separation from parents is unavoidable.

这就是我之前在第一章提到的，有时候想帮忙的人也会被拉进心理疾病的激流里面。看到所爱的人在激流中几乎要溺死的样子，虽然非常痛苦，但要永远记住：你自己也溺死的话，就无法帮助别人了。你必须设法保护你自己的精神及身体的健康。谦卑之石一直都在那儿，在你所爱的人（患者）找到它之前，他（她）很可能无法体会你所受到的痛苦，并且没办法接受你冒着那么大的风险而伸出的援手。很可惜的是，有些人就是要沉到心理疾病之河的最深处，才会承认他们需要别人的协助。我自己就是这样。事实上，当我沉到河里最深处时，还开始往河底的泥土挖洞！有好几年的时间，我的父母、家人及朋友只能远远地痛心地看着我，不知道在我明白使我生活状况越陷越糟的元凶就是自己之前，我还要挖那个洞到多深的地步。

This is what I was talking aboutin chapter one when I said others trying to help sometimes get pulled into the mental illness rapids themselves. As hard as it is to see your loved one drowning in the mental illness rapids, always remember this: You can't help another if you are drowning yourself. Do what you must to save your own sanity and health. Rock Humility is always there. Until your loved one finds it, he or she will probably be blind to your suffering and unable to receive the help you are risking so much to give. Sadly, some people have to sink to the very bottom of the "bipolar river" before they will admit they need help. I was this way. In fact, when I dropped to the bottom of the river, I started digging a hole in the mud! For years my parents, family and friends could only watch from a distance and painfully wonder how deep of a pit I would dig for myself before I realized I was only getting lower and lower.

不愿意承认疾病进入我的生活，就像是一个盲目的人一心想揭晓魔鬼用叱责般声音发出的谜语："你愿意挖多深的洞到达天堂呢？"当我想独力破解这道死题时，我一点一点、一铲一铲地把洞越挖越大，直到一头栽进我所知最险恶的火海。就在那时——当我的心被魔鬼的三尖叉刺透，然后放到火上当成串烧的时候，我终于看见自身的迷惑，开始承认自己有病，并且相信并接受爱我之人的建议与协助。在地狱烤肉炉上最惨痛的一次经验，就是在我向所爱的女孩求婚遭拒的时候。我不确定是不是因为我固执地不承认自己有病，她才拒绝我的求婚，但我的确知道我离开她去台湾之前，她曾写给我许多短笺和信，其中流露出对我深重而绵长的爱意。

Not authorizing my illness into my life was like being blindly obsessed with uncovering the answer to the devil's chiding riddle："How deep are you willing to dig to reach heaven?" While meddling with this mystery all alone, I picked, shoveled, and burrowed until I plunged headfirst into the worst flaming inferno I could imagine. It wasn't until then, when the devil's spike shish kebabbed my heart and held it over the fire, that I finally began to see my own confusion and start to authorize myself as someone with an illness who needed to trust and receive help from those who loved me. My incident, in purgatory's deepest barbeque pit, was a rejected proposal for marriage from the girl I loved. I don't know for sure if she said no because of the poor way I was handling my illness. I do know that before I left for Taiwan she had written dozens of notes and letters expressing deep and lasting love.

　　如果每次跟她亲吻就有人给我20美金的话，那么我现在已经是百万富翁了。甚至有一次她还问我，将来我们要生几个小孩，但自我在台湾和蒙大拿躁狂症发作之后，这种种热烈爱情的表现就跟国庆烟火秀最后一发烟火施放后一样——燃烧殆尽，变成缕缕灰烟，然后静静飘散消逝。当她说出"我不能"，拒绝我的求婚的那个伤心日之后，我终于停止否认我的疾病，开始承认这疾病就存在我的生活里。我再也无法蒙骗，装模作样地告诉自己"我很好，问题都在别人身上"。我的病烧毁了我一生中最大的目标，而我无法藏起那烫焦的伤疤。从那时起我再也没有否认现实，终于开始开放、坦诚地跟别人谈"我的病"。令我惊讶的是，当我跟别人诚实地说起有关我疾病的种种，他们的回应是理解、包容和爱，没有人把我当作是脆弱的怪胎，或是个疯狂的窝囊废；没有人开我的玩笑，或是在背后酸溜溜地讽刺我。

　　Also, if her kisses were twenties, I was a millionaire. Once, she had even asked me how many children I would like in our family. After my manic psychosis episodes in Taiwan and Montana all of these exploding expressions of love burned out and drifted away like silent wisps of gray smoke after the grand finale of a Fourth of July fireworks show. After she said "I can't" to my desperate marriage proposal on that devastating day, I finally stopped denying my illness and started authorizing it into my life. Telling myself I was fine and that everyone else had the problem was a front I couldn't fake anymore. My illness had charred my life's greatest goal and I couldn't hide the burn marks. From that point on, there was no denial of reality and I finally began to talk openly about my illness. The thing that surprised me was when I started honestly talking to people about my illness, they responded with understanding, tolerance, and love. No one thought I was a fragile freak, or treated me like a whacked-out wimp. No one cracked crude jokes or spewed sour sarcasm behind my back.

随着时间的流逝，我有了很神奇的发现：当我跟一些在生活上颇有成就的人和我很尊敬的人谈到我的病时，他们大多会告诉我他们自己或是他们认识的人也患有某种类型的心理疾病。我看到这些人虽然必须依靠药物治疗，但他们依然备受关爱；他们即使患了心理疾病也受到他人的尊敬，所以我想，也许我也能依靠药物的治疗，并同时保有他人的爱与尊重。当有那些真心在身边关心我的人拉我一把，帮助我从自己已挖了多年的洞中爬出来，我慢慢地开始了解，承认心理疾病的存在并不会使我变得软弱、没价值，或是变得怪异。我也学习到，让别人在我力不从心时帮助我，是很恰当、很好，甚至可以说是很健康的事。关爱我的人在听到我向他们寻求帮助的时候，总觉得那比看到我逞强、假装自己十全十美的样子要好多了。

As time went on and I spoke with high achievers and people I looked up to about my illness, it was amazing to discover that most of them either suffered from some type of mental illness themselves, or knew someone who did. When I saw how they were loved despite their dependence on pills or how they respected others despite mental illness, I thought that perhaps I could be dependent on medication and still be loved and respected, too. With the caring assistance of those around me lifting me up out of the hole I had dug for so many years, I slowly started to realize authorizing mental illness into my life did not make me weak, unworthy, or weird. I learned it is okay, good, and even healthy to allow others to assist me when I couldn't help myself. People who loved me thought better of me when I asked for needed help than when I pretended to be perfect.

　　事实上，假装自己没有任何弱点或病症其实是让我与别人变得更疏远，因为那样的我看来并不真诚。接受心理疾病进入我的生活的事实，就好像把一根大木柱从我眼中拔出来，也让我清楚地了解每个人都有其难处和弱点。承认患病，让我停止往下跌，并转而开始往上爬，也帮我敞开心扉，让他人来帮助、安慰我伤痛的心，修补我混乱的脑袋，让我能抓住他们伸出的引导之手。在盲目的状态下用信心跳跃——从第一块的"察觉"踏脚石跳到第二块踏脚石"承认"上，真的让我睁开眼睛，并使我看清我对这一疾病……还有对我自己的认识是多么浅薄。就好像我有一次去湖边钓鱼，我的钓鱼线在湖水里被另一条钓线缠上——它的主人在某处将纠结的它剪掉抛弃，把问题留给我——一样，我的心理疾病：躁郁症和我的个性混在一起，非常难以解开。只有仔细地检查及透彻的理解力才能帮上忙。

The truth was that acting like I didn't have weakness or illness actually distanced me from others because I didn't seem real or genuine. Authorizing mental illness into my life was like yanking two-by-fours out of my eyes. It helped me to clearly see that everyone else also carries crosses. It allowed me to stop falling down and start climbing up. And it opened my soul so that others could come in to help soothe my scalded heart, mend my mangled mind, and offer a guiding hand. Taking the blind leap-of-faith from the stepping-stone "Identify" to the eye opening "Authorize," allowed me to clearly see just how little I knew about my illness…and myself. Just like the time my fishing line tangled with the snagged up line of someone who had sliced his line and split, my mental illness: bipolar disorder, and my personality had become interwoven, knotted and difficult to work with. Only close examination and clear understanding could help.

于是在"承认"之后，我站在心理疾病的激流中，可以看到下一块叫作"明白"的踏脚石，它大到足以让我坐下，然后进行将我纠结的自我与疾病分开来的工作。

Standing in the mental illness rapids on "Authorize," I could see the next stepping stone, "Understand," was big enough for me to sit down and start untangling myself and my illness.

第四章 步骤三：明白你的疾病和你自己

我不是"神经病"
我是"患了心理疾病"的人

现在你应该能看得出来我喜爱钓鱼。涉水走过晶亮的小溪或乘船在透明的湖上钓狡猾的鳟鱼，对我而言都是天堂般的感受。也许，现实的心理疾病不能在我化学作用翻腾的脑海里将我对钓鱼的喜爱淹没，是因为我感觉在钓鱼时拥有的智慧和能力，似乎使我比平日更接近创造万物的慈悲老天爷。我不能钓鱼时，也喜欢写写有关钓鱼的事，我可以做出很多在生活跟钓鱼两者之间的分析和比较。在上一章的结尾，我已经用一个钓鱼经验（缠住的钓线）来比喻在生活中辨别心理疾病——为了分辨"明白"，我想继续来处理那几条缠住的"线"。

Chapter 4   Step Three: Understand
Your Illness and Yourself

I am not "mental illness"

I have mental illness

You can probably tell by now that I love to fish. To me, there is something heavenly about wading in a sparkling stream or floating on a crystal lake catching that cunning trout. Perhaps the reason mental illness can't drown away this love in the unbalanced river of my brain's chemistry is because I feel so close to the Master Fisher while doing it. When I can't fish, I like to write about fishing. There are so many analogies and comparisons I can make between life and fishing. I finished the last chapter, authorizing mental illness into my life, with a fishing metaphor. To discuss "Understand." I would like to continue casting those lines.

有时候我在钓鱼，钓线会被另外一条乱七八糟的渔线绞住。有些钓客在他们的钓线这样缠乱时，他们不愿意花时间弄好它，宁可剪下线赶快闪人。我不喜欢这样，我希望自己不是那种剪了线而让下一位钓客缠上麻烦的人，何况鱼钩和飞镖所费不赀，我也不想把它们抛弃掉。不过从混在一起的渔线中救出鱼钩来，常常不是一个简单的过程。有的时候线团复杂无比而且往往绞得很紧，光用拆的办法不可能处理妥善。最好的方法就是把不属于自己的线一段一段地剪开——心理疾病就很像这些外来的混乱钓线。当我本身跟这个病混在一起时，很难分别哪个是好线（自己）、哪个是乱线（心理疾病）。我的个性、习惯、情绪，甚至概念，都和我的疾病：躁郁症混乱交织在一起。

Often while fishing, my line gets tangled up in the mangled mess of another line. It's frustrating to become the victim of other fishers who, rather than untangle their snagged-up lines, simply cut them off and move on. I'm not the kind of person who can just clip my line and leave an even bigger mess for the next guy to tangle with. Besides, I pay good money for my flies and lures. I don't like to leave them behind. Saving them from the tangled mess can be tricky. Sometimes the twisted and tied knots are too complex and too tight to just unweave. The best way to fix these tangles is to clip away pieces of the line that isn't mine. Mental illness is a lot like that intruding line. When I got tangled up in it, it became very difficult to tell which was the good line (me) and which was the broken one (the disorder). My personality, habits, moods, and even beliefs all became mixed and meshed with my mental illness: bipolar disorder.

　　一开始我根本没想到可能是二条不同的"线"在催动或影响我，当时我以为这一团糟糕的生活都是命运带来的。多年来我一直否认这一团乱的严重问题，不愿意去研究并了解它。这就像把纠结的渔线乱扯乱拉，期望鱼线会自动理好，然而却将更多的纠结缠到我本来的人格上，时间一久，那些原有问题的症结也就越扯越紧。为了明白如何把自己跟躁郁症分开来，我必须回过头，看看自己躁狂症发作还有住院之前，也就是鱼线还是正常、纠结还不明显的那段日子。回首过往，我发现我的躁狂症首次出现的状况之一，是在我十几岁时不断绕着田径场跑步的时候。孩提至青少年时代的我，个性好强爱竞争，我喜欢胜过别人，若是输了就会号啕大哭。

At first I didn't think there were two separate "lines" of motivation or influence. I believed it was all one tangle; "just me, the way fate made me." For years I denied the seriousness of my snarl and refused to study and understand it. This was like yanking and jerking on my jumbled line, hoping to get an easy fix. All it did was tie more knots into my own personality that, over the years, tightened with each manic-depressive tug. In order to understand how to separate myself from my bipolar disorder I had to look back before the breakdowns and hospitals when the loops were loose and the knots were simple. In my past, I found that one of my first meshings with mania began in my mid-teens as I sprinted around and around the running track. As a child and teenager, I always had a competitive personality. I loved to win and bawled when I lost.

读高中时，我听过来自教练们及运动高手们许多鼓舞人的话："你什么都能做到""天空才是极限""唯一能限制你的就是你给自己的限制""设立目标、努力前进，你就可以达到任何高度"。这些鼓舞人的话语激励了我，天真的个性加上对胜利的强烈渴望，使我开始相信自己真的"无所不能"。在这种心态下，高三的我开始计划成为犹他州史上跑得最快的一英哩赛跑选手。那时候我全心全意地认为，只要够努力，我可以在那一季的比赛里每次都进步二秒。按照我心中的这个计划，在年底我会成为在犹他州一英里赛跑里打破四分钟记录的首位高中生——别梦想了，当时的我其实连五分钟跑一英里的纪录都还未打破。

During my high school years I heard a plethora of pep talks from coaches and successful athletes who said, "You can do anything." "The sky is the limit." "The only limitations you have are the limitations you put on yourself." "You can reach any height if you set a goal and climb hard enough." Their pep talks andclichés excited my mind. With my believing personality and tremendous desire for moments in the fleeting flicker of victory, I became convinced I could do *anything*. With this in mind, I came up with a plan my senior year to be the fastest high school miler in Utah's history. I honestly thought if I worked hard enough, I could take two seconds off each race through the season. I mapped out that by the end of the year, I would be the first high school student in Utah to break the four-minute mile. Forget that, up until then, I hadn't broken a *five*-minute mile.

　　到了年底，我最快的时间是四分四十二秒，还差十秒才能得到参加犹他全州比赛的资格。虽然教练们和父母都赞美说我那年做得很棒，田径的队友们签名在我的纪念册时，很多人写到他们对我的敬佩，因为当别的选手训练结束时，我还留在跑道上额外训练，然而我心里却不能认同这些赞美，反倒因为无法完成目标，觉得自己是个输家。这种沮丧感就像黄色警示带，我应该站在线外，专注于那些赞美，并为我已达到的进步而高兴，而不是蒙住眼睛和耳朵，一心相信更多的努力及更大的渴望可以让我达到我内心的超级目标。结果在跨越"警戒线"之后，就是我的人格与躁狂症开始交缠不清的危险起点。

At the end of the year, my fastest time was four minutes and 43 seconds; ten seconds short of even qualifying for the state meet. My parents and coaches all complimented me on a great season. Teammates signed my yearbook saying they looked up to me because I had run extra laps when everyone else had quit. Inwardly, I wouldn't accept praise. I felt like a failure because I missed my goal. These feelings of failure were like yellow caution tape. I should have stayed behind the line by paying attention to the compliments I received and being happy with the great improvements I made. Instead, I covered my eyes and ears with the belief that harder work and deeper desire could have brought to pass my grandiose goal. Crossing the "warning line" was a dangerous point when my personality began to mix with mania.

　　不久之后，当我搭飞机到中国台湾参加志愿服务时，完全没有人，甚至能闻出炸弹的嗅探犬，都无法侦测到我打包到台湾地区的"精神病炸弹"——那尚未被察觉的、易燃的爆炸性组合，就是以为自己是超人的自我期望，和日渐成形的躁狂症。我在台湾地区的十个月里，这两种危险成分混在一起，闪着"危险"警讯的烟雾开始使我自己和别人都感到窒息难过。因为饮食不正常、睡眠不足，也没有好好花时间去运动或放松，我的身体变得虚弱而且举止怪异。种种钻牛角尖的怪异思维歪曲了我头脑里面的现实，人们在跟我谈话的时候，越来越觉得我奇怪。当我的同事和朋友试着分摊我的工作分量，但都被我拒绝，惹我生气，我简直像一只高举尾巴的臭鼬一样无法亲近。

　　A short time later, when I boarded the plane and left for my volunteer service in Taiwan area, no one, not even bomb‑sniffing dogs, could detect a whiff of the mental explosives I packed along. The unidentified, combustible combination was superman self‑expectations and maturing mania. During my ten months in Taiwan area, as these two dangerous ingredients mixed together, smoking symptoms that should have set off flashing DANGER alarms started choking me and others around me. My body became weak and wired from a poor diet, lack of sleep, and not taking time to exercise or unwind. Deep, over‑focused obsessions warped my mind's reality and made me seem weirder and weirder to those I spoke with. When colleagues and friends tried to offer assistance with my workload, denial and irritability made me as approachable as a skunk with his tail raised.

我盲目地相信自己"只要努力，就能克服一切"，完全忽视所有的警讯，一步步地踏入危险的红色警戒区。就这样，我那"不可能的目标"的热度，猛烈的工作习惯，以及强迫性的思想，点燃了"躁狂症的火药"，导致我躁狂症炸弹的首度爆炸。

另一个由于个性跟躁郁症缠缠不清的例子，就是我的高三生活嘶嘶地冒出火花。那年我谈了恋爱；频繁的情书往来、晚间为了秘密会面而偷偷溜出家门，彻夜地在收音机和营火旁慢慢跳舞，我的心情比七月国庆日的烟火更高更热。当时我并未察觉异状，但两人一起创造回忆时，情感之波涛翻腾的力度，确实远超过了"正常"的底线。

年轻人的恋爱珍贵又强烈，不过对我而言，它跟隐藏难明的躁郁症混合在一起，其造成的负面影响持续之久，仿佛原子弹轰炸过后久久不散的核灾辐射。

I was so blinded by the belief I could work myself out of anything, I ignored all these warning signs and marched right into the bipolar red zone. There, the heat of my impossible goals, furious work habits, and obsessive thinking sparked the gunpowder of bipolar mania and set off the bomb of my first breakdown. Another dangerous combination of personality and bipolar disorder also started sparking and sizzling my senior year in high school. It was the year I fell in love. Sending and receiving love notes, sneaking out at night for secret rendezvous, and dancing the night away next to a boom box and campfire made me feel higher and hotter than bottle rockets in July. I didn't realize it then, but the intensity of emotion I felt as we made memories together shot high above "normal." Young love is precious and powerful. For me however, when combined with misunderstood bipolar disorder, the long-term effect was like nuclear fallout.

这种精神上的爆炸让我飞上云端，然而接着抗精神病的药物就浇灭我的心情，把我拉回现实，于是我已经生病的脑袋只能得出这一结论："如果我能再次跟我的高中女友在一起，我就能再次感受到那种快乐得飘飘然的心情。"当时的我不明白，我那"发展中"的躁狂症正在我和女友开心约会、情绪高涨的几个月中快速地成长；而现在，服用那些能让我的情绪高度下降到和大部分"正常"人相同状态的药物，让我感到我过剩的感性和热情从我的个性中被硬生生地抢走了。所以我与其寻求专业的精神病医疗，宁可花费心力，专注且拼命地尝试回到过去的"那段美好时光"——因为我对自己的病这样的误解，而开启了一连串的连锁反应，让我的生活开始纠缠打结。第一个（打不开的）死结就是相信我高中的甜心女友能重新带给我快乐。

After psychosis blasted me out of the clouds and antipsychotic pills doused me with reality, my cancerous reaction could only conclude, "I will feel happy and high again if I can just get back together with my high school sweetheart." I didn't understand developing mania had amplified, by many times, the high during those dating months. Now, taking medication that lowered me to the same level as most "healthy" folks made me feel disabled, as if the excess of emotion and passion had been amputated from my personality. Instead of seeking help for my mental health, I focused my efforts and attention on desperately trying to return to "how it was before." Misunderstanding the illness in this way started a chain reaction of knots and tangles in my life. The first knot (NOT) was believing my high school sweetheart could restore happiness.

当她在欧洲念书时，我每个月、每个星期、每天、每小时、每分每秒都在倒数直到她回家。如此不可思议的期盼与渴望之下，你必能想象当发现她已经不再爱我时，我有多么沮丧；而看到她嫁给另一位男子，那种痛苦让我感觉一切找回过往快乐的机会都永远地与我隔绝了。

"我的心被炸得粉碎""只能飞回台湾地区来找回失去的快乐"的念头，是另一个混乱的结。因此我让自己的生活被所有能找到属于华人文化的东西包围——在大学里与说中文的同学混在一起，自制印有中文的T恤，听中国的音乐，我用中文录音和写信，然后寄给在中国台湾的朋友们，选修中文课，跟华人女孩约会。我的所思所言全都是"假若有一天能回到台湾地区，我该会何等的快乐！"

While she studied abroad in Europe, I counted down each month, week, day, hour, and minute until she arrived home. With such incredible anticipation, you can imagine how devastating it was to discover she didn't love me anymore. The pain of seeing her marry another man felt like a divorce from any chance for the blessed bliss of the past.

The next knot of confusion came by concluding my heart had been bombed and I could only find happiness by evacuating back to Taiwan area. So, I surrounded myself with everything Chinese. I hung out with Chinese students at the university. I made T – shirts with Chinese writing on them. I listened to Chinese music. I sent tapes and wrote letters to friends in Taiwan area. I took Chinese classes and dated Chinese girls. All I could think and talk about was how happy I would be when I could return.

　　然而当我慈爱大方的父亲真的带我回中国台湾时，让我很困惑和沮丧的是，不到几天，那极度的高兴便消失了，抑郁又捕获了我，我一心只想回家。返家后的我，再度漫无头绪地想寻回年少时的那种狂喜（或者是说，那种躁狂脱序的飘然快感）。虽然斗牛比赛、赛跑还有滑水都是有趣的活动，却不再让我兴奋如前；把以前最爱的音乐放到很大声也只会让我心痛，就算头发留成80年代流行的长度也丝毫安慰不了我。好几年后我才开始了解并明白，在第一次病症爆发之前那种种强烈的快乐，都只是因为潜藏的躁郁症在作祟，而不是因为女孩，不是因为中国台湾小岛，也不是因为那个年代。慢慢明白事实的我，便渐渐能把真实的自己从过去混乱的线团里切割出来，开始接受一种不那么亢奋，但确实更加安稳的日常生活。

When my gracious and generous father took me on a trip back to Chinese Taiwan, it was confusing and frustrating that after just a few days, the high left, depression found me, and all I wanted to do was go home. When I got home, I continued running in circles searching for the bliss (or in other words, the manic highs) of my youth. Basketball pick-up games, road races, and waterskiing were fun, but not the "rush" they had been in the past. Cranking up my old tunes only gave me heartache. Even growing out the old '80s mullet hairstyle didn't help. It took many years to finally figure out and understand it was bipolar mania, and not the girl, the island, or the decade that made life seem so intensely wonderful before the manic psychosis breakdowns. As this understanding gently settled on my mind, I was able to cut myself away from the tangled line of the past and accept a lower but more stable level of daily living.

虽然我开始学会如何从受躁狂症影响的记忆纠结中分析出真实的自我，但在眼前还有一团难缠的乱丝要拆解，那就是难以分辨"难过"和"抑郁（症）"、"快乐"和"躁狂（症）"的差别。

当时我认为唯一能影响我的情绪的，是我的行为、环境还有心态，而不是我身体里面的化学成分。那时我知道伤害别人、撒谎、偷窃或类似的不好行为会使人感到难过，我也曾被教导过自愿扫地、送食物给需要的人，还有尽量服从道德的律法，是让人能体会真正快乐的法则。然而我不明白的是，为何为他人志愿服务或在晨间祈祷时我并不感到快乐，反而会忽然感到消沉与悲哀。在我内心的争战是，当我在深夜里研读与讨论的狂热情绪时，反而导致我入院，被人逼着睡觉、打镇静剂。被我曲解的躁郁症所带来的困惑非常真实而且复杂。

Even with an understanding of how to untie myself from mania-enhanced memories, there was still another sticky snarl to deal with. The next tightly tangled knot was misunderstanding the difference between sadness and depression and between happiness and mania. I believed emotions could only be influenced by my actions, my environment, and my attitude; not by chemicals in my body. I knew that hurting people, lying, steeling, or doing bad things caused sadness. I had also been taught that sweeping the floor without being asked, giving food to the hungry, and in general following moral laws was the way to feel true happiness. It didn't make sense that I felt down and blue while serving others or saying prayers in the morning. It baffled my mind that late at night, instead of enlightenment, my way up, superman high during moral book readings and spiritual discussions only led to emergency rooms and sedative injections. This confusing tangle of misunderstood bipolar disorder was very real and complex.

我可以了解为什么有那么多人被躁郁症所困，不约而同地养成上瘾、自我毁灭，自我挫败，甚至是犯罪的行为——因为他们根本不晓得或是不明白，到底他们的身体与心理发生了什么事。这样的误解让患病者开始以为，世上恒定的道德规则（做好事带来快乐，犯坏事则等同悲伤）并不适用于他们。然而这些规则确实适用在他们身上，问题是他们还不明白"难过"和"抑郁（症）"、"快乐"和"躁狂（症）"的区别在哪。再者，若有人说："我有躁郁症，所以在道德的种种律法中我是例外者，也因此我不必去服从。"这不是个有用的借口，因为躁郁症并不会迫使人们去过这样的生活。

I can see why so many others who get tangled up similarly fall into addictive, self‐destructive, self‐defeating, and sometimes even criminal behaviors. They simply don't know or don't *understand* what is happening in their bodies and minds. Misunderstanding the illness in this way can make people who suffer with it believe that moral rules (doing good brings happiness, doing bad equals sadness) don't apply to them. The truth is that these laws do apply to them; they just haven't yet learned the difference between depression and sadness and between mania and happiness. Furthermore, saying, "Since I have bipolar disorder I am an exception to moral rules, and therefore don't have to follow them," is not a valid excuse because the illness doesn't force them to live any certain way.

在我和躁郁症共同生活的许多年里，除了最狂躁的几个小时以外，它从未抢走我自由选择行为的能力。就算当我用药失衡、不明白为何在我做正义的事情使人感到沉闷的时候，我还是没有失去可以清清白白、问心无愧地过生活的选择能力。当时我已是可以合法饮酒的年龄，我搬离了父母的家，一个人住在外面的公寓，只要我愿意，我可以追求色情、毒品，或者和酒吧里认识的女孩们有一夜情。即使当时我停止念书，也没有人会介意。我可以很容易地用疾病做借口，远离原来的高道德标准。然而问题是我不可能这样做，因为高道德标准是那能够让我得到真实而恒久快乐的"钩子"——一个绑住我混乱缠结的钩。

In all my years of living with this illness, except for the few hours during my most extreme psychotic episodes, bipolar disorder has never stolen my ability to choose my actions. Even when I didn't have balanced medication and didn't understand why I felt depressed doing spiritual things, I never lost the ability and freedom to choose a life that kept me with a clean slate and clear conscience. I was old enough to drink. I moved away from my parents into an apartment where I could have sought relief from pornographic flicks, flings with illegal drugs, and one-night-stands with girls from local bars. No one would have said anything if I stopped going to school. It would have been very easy to seek for instant relief by cutting my own line and using my illness as an excuse to walk away from my high moral standards. The problem with doing this, however, was that "high moral standards" was the hook I needed to catch true and lasting happiness—and it was the hook tied to the end of my tangled line.

在我的脑袋被这些乱糟糟的纠结所混乱的时期，我一直认为单单"行善"绝不可能是医治抑郁的良药——有股黑暗的疑云开始笼罩着我的信心，一个嘲弄的声音在我的脑海中，像是在引诱着我："如果你依照你观念中所教导的原则做好事、过正义的生活，却感觉不到'快乐'，也许你的神并不存在！"就像一个在洪水中快要淹死的人，对救难人员大喊着"不用过来！神会救我！"然后拒绝抓住他人的援手爬上救生船，我从未想过现代的药物可能就是我一直等待着的、来自上天的礼物。在这样沮丧低迷的黑雾之中，我必须做个选择："我到底要不要继续坚持我的行善生活？即使那样做似乎不会让我比较快乐？"我花了很长的时间思考这个问题，最后我决定不要放弃——在某天晚上，在我快要写完一篇很长、很悲伤的日记时，我写出了这个句子："虽然现在我感觉不到神存在我生命里，但是我无论如何都要继续跟随他！"

During this time of confusion with the snarled knot in my brain so set on believing that only "goodness," not pills, could help with depression, the darkness of doubt started clouding out my faith. A taunting voice in my mind tempted, "If righteous living doesn't make you 'happy' like your faith says it should, maybe God doesn't exist." Like the drowning flood victim who yelled out, "No thanks, heaven will save me," and then refused to grasp a helping hand and climb into a life boat, I didn't consider that modern medication could actually be the Divine gift I was waiting for. In these dark mists of depression, I had to make a choice: "Do I continue to live my faith even though it doesn't seem to make a difference in my happiness?" It took a lot of soul searching, but I decided not to give up. In conclusion to a long, depressed entry in my journal one night, I wrote, "I don't feel God in my life now. But I choose to follow Him anyway."

尽管脑筋弄不明白我情绪的起伏，但我内心深处知道，我需要寻求帮助，从内心寻找问题的症结。生活在无知的黑暗中，我感觉自己处在永远的长夜里。不过就跟老天爷必定不会放弃那些不放弃他的人一样，破晓灿烂的朝晖终究会射进我的世界。当我继续过着正义的生活，认识了一位美丽又聪慧过人的年轻女子，她当时跟我一样，正在寻找一个同样具有高道德价值观的配偶。连我告诉她我在精神方面的病历时，她也不为所动，继续培养我们的关系。有趣的是，和她缔"结"连理竟成为大大地帮助我脱离躁郁症这个与我纠缠不清的"结"的最大帮助。我不要让你有所误解，以为当我们在婚礼上说"我愿意"的时候所有的躁郁症问题都解决了。婚姻并不容易，就算对健康正常的夫妇来讲亦是如此，而我的心理疾病经常使我们要面对的挑战比常人更大。

Despite misunderstanding my highs and lows, deep inside I knew I should continue to look upward for help and inward to find the problem. Living in misunderstood darkness felt like a long black night. But, as it always does for those who do not give up on their Heavenly Father, eventually the sunshine of a new day brightened my world. As I continued to live as I should, I met a beautiful and talented young woman. She was searching for a husband who had the same high moral values she did. Even when I slipped her an honest "mental illness disclaimer," she still felt good about pursuing a relationship with me. How ironic that the blessing of "tying the knot," turned out to be the biggest help in untangling myself from my bipolar disorder. Now, I don't want to give the impression that marriage untangled everything the minute we said, "I do," or that marriage is the "cure all" for everyone with bipolar disorder or any other mental illness. Marriage is tough, even for healthy folks.

　　结婚后没多久，有时抑郁的情况严重到让我只能躺在床上哭个不停，这时我的妻子会坐在我身旁，握着我的手并轻柔地哼着充满希望的歌。我相信有段时间，她必定在怀疑我有没有办法让自己从心理疾病的病情中解脱。她从来没有放弃。因为我自己不愿意去做，所以她为我订购我该吃的处方药，并把药准备好、放在我会注意到的地方。她从不提醒或逼迫我吃药，但渐渐地，我越来越相信她的爱和忠诚一如在婚礼上的誓约，我有了勇气，也开始吃她为我留在盥洗台上的药。逐渐地，当明朗与快乐像阳光般慢慢照亮了我的生活，驱散我黑暗而绝望的抑郁时，我了解到这不是单纯因药效得到的收获——药物只是帮助我从疾病中松绑，让我能在应该快乐的时候感到欢喜，在应该悲伤的时候觉得难过。在这道新的曙光中，我可以清楚看见我所遵行的道德法则都是真实的。

My mental illness often magnified the challenges we faced. Early on, sometimes depression hit me so hard all I could do was lie on the bed crying. My wife, Sariah, sat with me during those times, holding my hand and softly singing hymns of hope. For a while, I'm sure she wondered if I would ever separate myself from my disorder. She never gave up. Because I wouldn't, she called in my prescriptions, picked them up, and kept them where I could see them. She never prodded or pushed me to take them. As I came to trust her love and commitment, I found the courage to take the pills she left on the counter for me. Slowly, as bright happiness shone away much of my dark depression, I came to the understanding that the pills didn't force it on me. Rather they simply loosened me from my illness and allowed me to feel happy (or sad) when I should. In this new light, I could clearly see the moral laws that I believed in and that I stuck with were true.

即使我正处于躁狂状态的激烈兴奋感里，犯罪其实换不来幸福。如果我做错什么，治疗抑郁的药不能治愈后悔与心痛。然而美德、正义、忠信、行善并服从道德的规定，却永远能为我带来平安。现在，正确的药让我开始感受到正义与善良带来的快乐。抗抑郁的药物是个大奇迹，但是它并没有完全医好我的病，如同抗狂躁的药只能把我调整到一个比较正常的亢奋高度，治疗抑郁的药物则是将我从危险的低谷拉升到接近正常的低处；药物的确将心理疾病所造成的乱结放松了，但它并没有让我完全脱离躁郁症。回到之前钓线的比喻，我接下来要谈的就是：为了使提供的帮助有效，病患的亲友们也要有意识地去理解患者脑中那堆打结的钓线，否则就算抱着一番好意，他们自己的钓线也可能会被卷进那团纠缠不清的混乱之中。

Committing crime never was happiness; even if I was on a manic high. If I did wrong, my antidepressant pills didn't take away the regret and pain. Virtue, uprightness, faithfulness, holiness, and following moral rules always brought peace, and now, the gift of correct medication allowed me to feel, to a degree, the resulting happiness. Antidepressant medications were a great miracle. However, they did not completely cure my depression. Just like the antipsychotic meds only brought me down to a more "normal" high, the antidepressant meds only lifted me up to a "normal" low. Medications helped loosen me from my tangle with mental illness, but they did not separate me completely from it. This brings me to my next point. In order to be effective help, friends and loved ones also must be willing to understand the tangled-up fishing line. Otherwise, despite good intentions, they might end up getting their own lines tangled in the mess.

让我举个自身的例子。当年我到中国台湾做志愿服务的头几个月里，也就是在我的躁狂症严重发作之前，我跟一位叫游南的年轻人成了朋友。在我发病并被送回美国后的十几年间，我们一直用口语录成带子彼此寄来寄去，以保持密切的联系；他所居住的台湾距离我身处的美国犹他州有半个地球之遥，但我一直觉得他就在我的身旁，陪伴我度过因躁狂症和抑郁症而感到最痛苦的时光。我曾寄给游南许多录音带——向他描述我的生活，以及躁郁症所带给我的痛苦，然而他对我的疾病的了解一直到我重回台湾拜访他的时候，他才切身地见识到实际的状况。一开始，能与游南重逢的兴奋之情让我无比雀跃，所以我一直笑容满面地跟他聊个没完；但过了三天之后，我的心情就像是收到海运送来摔坏的包裹那么的抑郁；好像只是一转眼，我的脸色就完全变了：我变得不想跟他说任何话。

For example, before my first manic psychosis breakdown and during my first few months of volunteer service in Chinese Taiwan, I made friends with a young man nicknamed "Yoner." After I returned home to the USA, we kept in close contact for over a decade sending voice tapes back and forth. He lived half a world away, but I felt like he was with me through the hardest times of depression and mania. Even though I had sent him hours and hours of voice tapes describing my life and struggles with this disorder, the reality of the illness never hit him until I took a trip back to Taiwan to visit him. At first, the excitement of being together with Yoner held me high and kept me chattering with a gleaming and interested smile on my face. Then, three days into the trip, like the arrival of a busted up, slow boat package, depression caught up to me. Almost instantly my whole countenance changed. Suddenly, I didn't have anything to talk to him about.

当我们在美丽的观光景点拍照时，面对镜头的我毫无笑意，一点白牙都不露；因为我一直拉长着脸且一言不发，游南开始怀疑自己是否做错了什么，或是不经意地冒犯了我，所以他的心充满了遗憾与后悔，换句话说，他的钓线已经被我那堆乱七八糟的线团缠住了。直到他向我道歉，说"我没有好好招待你"时，我才明白发生了什么事。我心痛地向他解释，说他并没有做错什么，我没有生他的气或有任何不满，只是我自己困在抑郁的循环里而已。游南很难理解我的态度会这样无缘无故地转变，但是他至少停止了自责。当我搭飞机回美国时，一直思考着游南对我在情绪和行为转变上的误解，并回想起过去的生活中，也有许多虽然抱持着好意却不明白个中缘由，因而被我混乱的精神所困缚的人们。

I couldn't even show teeth when he took photos of me at tourist spots we visited. With the long face and no talking, Yoner started thinking he had done something wrong or that he had offended me. Inside he felt horrible and guilty. In other words, he got tangled up in my messed up line. It wasn't until he apologized for "not taking good care of me," that I realized what was happening. With a heavy heart, I explained to him that he had done nothing wrong. I wasn't mad at him or anything like that. I was simply suffering from depression. Although it was hard for him to understand I could look and feel that way without any specific event or logical reason, at least he stopped blaming himself. While flying home from Taiwan, I pondered about Yoner's misunderstood reaction to my appearance and tone. I thought back on many different experiences in my life where well meaning, but ignorant people got tangled up in my mental mess.

我了解到，他们是因为"误会"而对我的感情表现和我需要的帮助做出了错误、甚至是完全相反的判断，这一发现让我几乎要落泪。接下来让我和你分享一些我所想到的回忆。有一天我睡了整整十二小时才起床，在下午一点钟脚步蹒跚地走进办公室。我的同事只看了我一眼，就对我说："你看起来好累，一定是工作得太过头了，赶快回家去睡个午觉吧！"还有一次，是在我的躁狂症即将发作——我得去医院接受注射才能安静下来——的前一晚，一位朋友告诉我，我的想法非常深奥而奇妙，她觉得我有无穷的精力，而且我有非常积极正面的能量，让她忍不住跟我一聊就聊到凌晨三点。有一回连工作的老板也误解了我的抑郁症状，那时我接到一个在大清早开会的任务，我诚实地说我担心自己无法及时起床开会，然而我最后还是说："但我愿意试试看。"

It was sadly comical to realize how "misunderstanding" made them assume exactly the opposite of what I was feeling and what kind of help I needed. Let me share some of the memories I thought about. One time, after sleeping for 12 hours, I stumbled into the office at 1：00 PM. Taking one look at my depressed face my coworker said, "You look so tired. You're working too hard. Go home and take a nap." Another time, the night before a manic breakdown forced me to a hospital where only injections could settle me down, a friend said my thoughts were deep and profound. She felt I had so much strength and so much positive energy she wouldn't stop talking to me until 3：00 AM. Yet another time, even my employer misinterpreted my depression. When I was given an assignment that required early morning meetings, I expressed honest concern that I might not be able to get out of bed in time. "But I'm willing to try." I concluded.

　　语毕，他盯了我一会儿，然后对我说："你知道在你原本说可能起不了床的时候，你的脸色黯淡无光，而当你说你愿意试试看的时候，你的脸色随即转亮了吗。就像现在我这样跟你讲话的时候，我觉得你的面容越来越有光彩了！"事实上，我的脸色"越来越有光彩"是因为我感到挫败和愤怒而产生的面红耳赤；他看到的黯淡表情是因我的抑郁所致，而不是他误以为的"因为懒惰而捏造了蹩脚借口"。说到借口，让我们与躁郁症患者的雇主或亲友谈谈"明白（躁郁症）"这个主题，父母跟位居领导阶层的人要面对的最大挑战之一，往往便是不管别人（孩子或下属）有什么疑问或借口，都要加以激励。然而，在与心理疾病的病患相处时这可能是件很危险的事，让我举个例子：

After watching me closely, one of the supervisors said, "Did you know your countenance was dark when you said you might not be able to get out of bed? Now I can see you are getting a light countenance as I tell you this." What I was actually feeling as "my countenance lightened" was red – faced anger and frustration. The "dark countenance" he had seen was simply depression, not a revelation of inner laziness covered by lame excuses. Speaking of excuses, let's discuss a very important "understand" issue regarding leaders and loved ones of people suffering from bipolar disorder. So often, one of the greatest challenges parents and people in leadership positions face is motivating others despite their doubts and excuses. This can be very dangerous when dealing with someone suffering from mental illness. Let me give a hypothetical example to explain:

　　有位老板在听到员工打电话来说"我今天生病，不能去上班"时，老板内心并不相信员工真的病了，所以他又劝又哄，讲了许多能说服员工来上班的"鼓励"的话，直到员工最后承认他那天其实只是想去滑雪。员工来上班时，老板自豪地觉得他成功了。同一天，另一位员工告诉老板他承受不了工作上的压力，想要比较轻松的任务。老板认为这也是个逃避工作的借口，就用同样的方式来应付，开始滔滔不绝，不停"鼓励"那位心中烦闷的员工，直到他答应继续做同样的工作为止。一个星期后，老板吃惊地听到那员工向工会申请了高昂的员工理赔，而且由于老板给她的压力，促成她的躁郁症发作而提出法律诉讼。

　　When an employer receives a phone call with the excuse，"I'm sick and can't come to work today." the boss feels inclined not to believe that the employee is really sick. So she pushes and coaxes until the employee finally admits he just wants to go skiing that day. When the employee shows up to work，the boss beams with the glow of success and accomplishment. That same day another employee tells the boss she needs a lighter work load because the stress is too much for her to handle. Thinking it is just another excuse to get out of work，the boss uses the same tactics she used on the employee who made excuses earlier. She talks，pushes，and "encourages" the stressed employee until she agrees to keep trying. A week later the boss is shocked to receive news of a hefty lost time workman's compensation claim along with the possibility of a personal law suit for forcing a manic psychotic episode on an employee who suffers from bipolar disorder.

补充说明：如果你以为，身为老板"只要不雇用任何有精神病的人就好。"要记住有百分之五十的躁郁患者是没有被确诊或遭到误诊的。换句话说，他们并不知道自己患病；即使他们知道，美国也有保护隐私的严格法律，好让这类资讯在求职面试与背景调查中永远秘密地锁在当事人心里。还有，当你看到今日在美国有那么多歧视案件的时候，可能也会改变想法——难道简单地学习这个疾病的种种，明白它，然后跟你的员工合作，不是容易得多吗？与患有躁郁症（或任何其他正式的心理疾病或障碍）的人交流时，父母、上司和公司老板都必须仔细倾听并严肃地面对我们所诉说的顾虑。但我也知道这会打开让"摸鱼""懒惰"进来的门，或者让抑郁症为所欲为。

Side note: If you are an employer who says, "I just won't hire anyone with mental illness." remember this: over 50% of people with bipolar disorder are undiagnosed or misdiagnosed. In other words, they don't even know they have it. Even if they do know, strict confidentiality laws keep this type of information securely locked away from job interviews and background checks. Also, take a look at all the discrimination cases out there and you might change your mind. Wouldn't it be easier to simply learn of the illness, come to understand it, and then work with your employee? When dealing with people who suffer from bipolar disorder (and any other legitimate illness or handicap) parents and leaders must listen carefully to our concerns and take them seriously. I know this opens the door to "slacking." being lazy, or perhaps even allowing depression to take control.

　　这就是为什么明白我们的疾病是那么重要。当你确实了解我们和我们的病，你就会知道何时应该加紧鼓励，何时则要松手让我们放松。我一次又一次地听到别人说"你看来很正常""你只要更努力就好""问题都来自你的心态"还有"只要乖乖吃你的药就没事了"之类的话，让我确信一般人对于躁郁症以及其他心理疾病仍有极大的误解。当人们真诚地关心我，懂得透过疾病的症状而了解我的本性，并且认为罹患心理疾病就像得了癌症、糖尿病或自闭症一样"正常"而真实，那是多么珍贵而美好的事啊！把我的疾病和真正的我分个明白，是我在脱离急流的过程中一块非常重要的踏脚石。在这个阶段，我找到了真正的我——是一位婚姻幸福、工作很努力、忠心且充满爱的丈夫和父亲，只是患了一种病。当我会没来由地感到自己很失败，内心失落，了无生趣，连做点简单的家事的动力都没有，不是一个真诚的朋友，甚至不配进天国……我知道那只是我的抑郁症在作祟。

This is why understanding our illness is so important. When you understand us and our illness, you will know when to push and when to back off. Hearing the ignorant words, "You look fine to me." "Just try harder." "It's all in your head." and "Just go take your meds." over and over again has convinced me that bipolar disorder and other mental illnesses are still greatly misunderstood. How precious and rare it is when others care enough to look beyond my appearance and understand that my illness is as "normal" and real as cancer, diabetes, or autism. "Understanding" my illness and me was a very important stepping-stone. There I found the real me. I was a happily married, hard working, dedicated, and loving husband and father tied to an illness. When, *for no reason*, I felt like a failure, sad, uninterested in life, lacking motivation to do simple tasks, not a true lover or friend, or unworthy for heaven, I knew it was only depression.

　　而在某些夜里，当我脑中的思绪奔腾，像要超越宇宙甚至永恒的边疆，因而无法入眠的时候，我知道那只是躁狂症发作的症状。此一认知让我能够与我的疾病分开，因为我知道那些症状都是暂时性且能被治疗的，它们不是我本有的个性。走上"明白"这块踏脚石，让我得以放松，并逐步剪断使我停滞不前的"躁郁乱线"，使我有办法收卷自己的钓线，"钓"到快乐的生活——我所需要做的只是继续"控制"剩下的部分就好了。是的，下一步，就是帮助我们屹立于心理疾病急流之上的"控制"。

　　When I couldn't sleep at night and my thoughts raced to eternity and beyond, I knew it was simply mania. This understanding separated me from my disorder because I knew the symptoms were temporary and treatable. They were not my permanent personality. Conquering the stepping-stone "Understand" allowed me to loosen and clip myself free enough to resume reeling in a happy life again! All I needed to do was *control* the knots that remained. "Control" turned out to be the next stepping-stone out of the mental illness rapids.

第五章　步骤四：控制你的疾病

我不能使河水停止流动

但我可以引导河水的流向

我喜爱奥运。看到世界各国齐聚一堂进行友善的体育竞赛，总让我的心中充满对世界和平的期望。其中我特别喜欢看的一项竞赛是体操，看着选手跳跃、旋转、翻身，让我联想到在空中飞来飞去的超级英雄们。但即使是奥运选手也不是完美无缺的，有时候体操选手会失去平衡、倾斜，甚至摔下。我记得在某天晚上的撑竿跳竞赛中，有一位实力强大、很有夺金希望的选手，他快速助跑到跳板位置，撑竿高高地跃上空中，在充满力道与优美的扭身翻转之后，他用双脚着地，但就在那一刻，他的身体有点失衡偏斜，虽然不致于跌倒，但他也不想踏出一步而破坏原本的落地姿势，于是他宁可挥动双臂来保持平衡。

Chapter 5　Step Four：Control Your Illness

I can't stop the river

I can direct its flow

I love the Olympics. Seeing the nations come together for friendly competition fills me with hope for a peaceful world. One venue I especially enjoy is gymnastics. Watching them spring, spin, tumble, and turn reminds me of superheroes flying through the air. But even Olympians are not perfect. Now and then, gymnasts lose their balance, waiver, and even fall. I remember one night in the vault competition one of the gold medal hopefuls did just that. He sprinted to the springboard and vaulted high into the air. After twisting and flipping with power and grace, he landed on both feet, but leaned just a little to the side. Rather than take a step to keep from falling, he flailed his arms in the air trying to catch his balance.

这让他的动作看来很滑稽，因为他看起来好像在跳小鸡舞（chicken dance），连他自己也尴尬地笑了；最后，他还是移动了脚步才避免跌倒。比赛中有两位评论员，其中一位也随着观众的反应开始笑起来，但是另一位觉得这并不好笑——他是一位曾获得奥运金牌的退休运动员，很了解比赛时裁判会注意的评分重点。他声音严肃地解说道："这小舞步般的动作可能会让这位选手失去金牌。"另一位评论员反驳："他的助跑、空中技巧和落地都几乎完美，一点点像是跳舞的脚步为什么会对他的分数有那么大的影响？"充满智慧的金牌评论员很有自信地回答："体操的精髓本来就在于控制。双手在空中乱摆和嬉笑等于告诉裁判：'我失去控制了，我很尴尬，因为我别无选择'。"

The action appeared almost comical, like he was doing the chicken dance, and he started laughing in embarrassment. He ended up still having to take the step to keep from falling. Along with the rest of the audience, one of the two commentators started laughing as well. The other commentator, however, didn't think it was funny. He was a retired Olympic gold medalist who understood what the judges watched for. With a serious voice he explained, "That little dance move may have cost him the gold medal." The other commentator objected, "His approach, aerial tricks, and landing were near perfect. Why would a little dance to catch his balance hurt his score?" The wise Olympic medalist commentator confidently replied, "Gymnastics is about control. Throwing your arms in the air and laughing about it tells the judges, 'I am out of control, and I'm embarrassed because there is nothing I can do about it.'"

即使跳马的动作很精彩，但他画蛇添足的姿势反而拉低了他的分数。果然，当成绩出现在计分板上，那位年轻的奥运选手确实因为"小鸡舞"而搞砸了夺牌的机会。

那段比赛的情况曾多次在我的脑海中盘旋，我会把自己比作那位倒霉的选手。躁郁症就好像是精神世界中的体操竞赛，能够好好控制情感和思绪的各种翻转、飞腾和降落，就意味着胜利与成功；如果没有控制好呢？嗯，我们都可以预料摔落在地的模样吧？我绝不是什么奥运体操高手，但我可以在弹簧床上做出后空翻动作。在这项运动中我学习到如何控制好自己和防止自己摔破脑袋的秘诀，那就是要保持平衡；失去平衡的同时，就会失去控制。"躁郁症"病如其名，就是一种很典型的"失去平衡"的病症。

Even though the vault was great, the dance is what stood out. It will hurt him more than if he had just taken a small controlled step. Sure enough, when the scores were revealed, the young Olympian had danced his way out of the competition.

That Olympic moment has tumbled through my mind many times. The reason I think about it so often is because I can relate to the unfortunate guy. Bipolar disorder is a lot like mental gymnastics. Controlling the flipping, flying, and falling thoughts and emotions means triumph and success. Not controlling them···well, we've all seen the crashes. I'm not by any means an Olympic gymnast. I can however, do back flips on a trampoline. I have learned the secret to keeping control, and to avoid crashing on my head, is balance. The minute I lose balance is the instant I lose control. Bipolar disorder, by its very name and nature, is the model of an out of balance illness.

　　许多世纪以来，患病者跟这个社会都试图攻克躁郁症，但总是不得要领。在一、两个世代之前，这一疾病让患者在亢奋的躁狂症和低迷的抑郁症之间不稳定地晃荡，而当时可知的唯一能控制发作病况的方式，就是叫穿着白色大褂的男护士来帮忙，将人带走并锁进保护机构——讲明白点，就是关进疯人院——那是患病者几十年来都会难以忘怀的一种耻辱。今日，感谢许多很棒的组织，例如全美心理疾病联盟（NAMI, National Alliance for the Mentally Ill）、抑郁症与躁郁症支持联盟（The Depression and Bipolar Support Alliance），因为他们的努力，这种以精神病为耻辱的社会现象，正慢慢地如云烟般散去。他们的网站（例如：www. nami. org，或是用网络搜寻"精神病"，就能查到许多有帮助的办法与通道）提供了清楚而崭新的观察、可信赖的现代研究成果、看诊介绍和技巧、危机热线，以及相关的支持团体。

For centuries, both the victim and society have teetered and tottered trying unsuccessfully to gain control of it. It was just a generation or two ago when this disorder still took victims to such unstable highs and lows, the only known way to regain control was to call the men in white coats. The indignity of being dragged away and locked up in secured institutions became a stigma that is taking decades to dispel. Today, thanks to wonderful organizations like NAMI (The National Alliance for the Mentally Ill), the Depression and Bipolar Support Alliance, and many others, the stench of mental illness stigma is slowly being blown out to the winds of yesterday. Their websites (NAMI. org, DBSAlliance. org, or internet search "mental illness" for hundreds of others) offer clean and fresh insight, respected research, counseling referrals and tips, crisis intervention, and support groups.

多亏这些团体、组织的热情付出，今天让精神病患者在一般社会中生活并有所贡献不再是疯狂的想法了。当我们睁开眼去了解精神病，会发觉它并不是那么难控制的东西，只不过是一种使患者失去"平衡"的生理疾病，如果患者能找回平衡，他们就能掌握控制。我并没有说躁郁症是可以痊愈的，而是说它是可以被控制的。虽然现在有友善的药房在卖进步的、奇迹般的药物，也有训练有素的专门人士愿意分享使人耳目一新的课程和有效的咨商，但是躁郁症并没有完全被克服。很多人不明白这一点，世上没有一颗魔术药丸，能让人一吃就立刻彻底地根治躁郁症。很多人以为只要精神病患者乖乖吃药，一切事情就会变得像甜甜圈，或糖果，或薄荷口香糖一样甜甜蜜蜜。

Thanks to their ambitious efforts, the thought of mentally ill people living and functioning in society is not such a *crazy* idea any more. Now as we charge at mental illness head on we are coming to realize it isn't such an out of control thing. It is simply a biological disorder that throws people off course. Balance them out, and once again you have control. Now, I didn't say bipolar disorder could be cured. I said it could be controlled. Even with friendly neighborhood pharmacies offering modern, miracle medications and well‐trained professionals sharing eye‐opening education and competent counseling, bipolar disorder is still not "in the bag." There is no magic pill that instantly and permanently eliminates the illness. Many people don't understand this. They think if mentally ill people would just take their medication, everything would be cookies, candy, and minty-fresh chewing gum.

事实上，要找到符合患者需求和个人特质的药物以及治疗方式，可能需要长达数月的时间来尝试错误。而且即使用药，抑郁与躁狂这两种"怪物"也不会被完全消灭，它们只是被锁在用昂贵的药品筑成的柱子上（我每天要吃的药丸好贵，而且许多保险公司的保险项目都不包含精神病药物！）当我站在"明白"这块踏脚石上，尝试找到通往下一块踏脚石——也就是"控制"——的时候，我注意到在我脚下潺潺的河水逐渐变得清晰。俯视着冒泡泡的水池，看见涟漪中自己的倒影，让我感到既新鲜又害怕：倒影中显示出一个善良、有能力，而且很能干的人，不过当我更仔细且深入地看着倒影，我看见的是一个永远会被精神病像黑暗而恐怖的阴影缠身的年轻人，这个阴影，只有在我熟睡时才不存在。

In actuality it may take months of trial and error to find the right combination of pills and personality adjustment. Once there, the monsters of depression and mania don't disappear. They are only chained up and held down with a costly chemical stake (My daily medication is so expensive! Also, many insurance companies won't cover psychiatric medicines!). As I stood on the stepping – stone "Understand," trying to figure out how to get to the next stepping – stone, "Control," I noticed the fizzing water beneath me had become clear. Looking into the bubbling pool and seeing my rippled reflection was refreshing and frightening at the same time. The reflection revealed a good, capable, and competent person. However, as I studied the reflection more deeply, I saw a young man with a mental illness permanently attached to him like a dark and scary shadow. It never left, except at night when I was asleep.

对事实的这一认知使我非常害怕，而且，非常令人……嗯，抑郁。我知道不能回到之前那灰暗的"无知"水域，我开始把注意力放在倒影中的暗影，而非那个开朗光明的人，这让我的情绪开始下沉到沮丧的深处。我觉得自己已经付出很多努力、走得这么远而来到这里，可是此时明白我的疾病状况，就像是逼我后退一步，并再度搅乱我的生活。仿佛我喝了一大口那因"明白"而清澈的水，以为会感受到清凉、畅快，但是却吞进了错误的管道。于是那些负面的想法开始从我溺水的脑袋中喷出来："明明知道今天提早起床去参加工作指派的教育研讨会，只会让我隔天抑郁得更厉害，为什么我还要去呢？""何必写诗、写故事，或做其他艺术创作？'灵感'只是我在夜晚躁狂症发作时瞬间出现的东西罢了。""我知道吃药会让我变胖，干吗还要运动？"

This part of understanding was very daunting and … well … depressing. Knowing I couldn't go back to the cloudy waters of ignorance, I started to focus more on the dark shadow in the reflection than on the bright person. This made me start to sink in despair. I felt I had come so far to reach this point. Now, understanding my illness seemed to take me back a step and choke up my life. It was like taking a big drink of the clear water, expecting cool refreshment, and swallowing it down the wrong tube. Choked up thoughts started spewing from my drowning brain. "Why get up early for education seminars at work when I know it will only result in enhanced depression the next day?" "Why write poetry, stories, or other creative things when I know the 'inspirations' are only fleeting, nighttime mania?" "Why exercise when I know my medication causes weight gain?"

"我知道抑郁症就是会叫我起床的闹钟，所以为什么需要早点上床？""当我知道那些热情的渴望都只是躁狂症作祟，为什么还要努力去跟别人做朋友？""为什么明知思考太多、太深就会让我精神病发作，我还得做那些让我充满压力的功课？"

一味执着于躁郁症会带来的必然症状，让我对追求品质更好的生活的渴望越来越少，我的心理疾病成为我动不动就拿来逃避事物的借口。然而后来，在一场三对三的篮球斗牛赛时，我被上了刻骨铭心的一课。当我在追球时，对方的一位球员冲撞我，使我的肩膀脱臼，即使肩膀骨头被推回原位，过了几分钟，我的手臂和手指仍然感到剧烈的痛楚。当我强忍疼痛喊着"犯规"时，那个家伙完全没有抗议——他是故意撞到我的。

"Why go to bed early when I know depression is my wakeup call?" "Why make efforts to keep friendships when I know the 'burning desire' is only mania?" "Why should I be required to do stressful homework when too much deep thinking can cause psychosis?" Over focusing on the inevitable inclusions of my mental illness tripped up my will to continue climbing toward a higher quality of life. My disorder became an *excuse* that was easy to hide behind. Then, while playing in a three-on-three basketball tournament, I received a hard-hitting, life lesson. While scrambling for a loose ball, one of the men on the other team knocked my shoulder out of its socket. Even after popping it back into joint for a minute or two, the intense pain still shot down my arm and into my fingers. In agony I hollered, "foul." The man didn't debate the call. He had hit me on purpose.

犯规暂停时间结束，当我再度面对他并准备发球时，我用另一只手护着我受伤的肩膀，期盼他因我的受伤而感到愧疚。然而事实与我期待的相反，他不但没有道歉的意思，还故意学我的样子抓住他自己的肩头，伴随着冷笑和挖苦我的表情，还发出小婴儿因尿布疹不适而哭闹的声音来嘲笑我。我彻底明白了：对手看到我受伤只会觉得高兴，而且如果还有机会让我胆怯和受挫的话，他一定会再次撞伤我。我看看我的队友们，他们很担心我，而且需要我。如果我选择躲在"因伤无法比赛"的借口背后并放弃努力的话，我就是在扯队友们的后腿，而让我们队伍输掉。我唯一能做的就是忍耐，并继续用我受伤的肩膀打完整场比赛。

When I checked him the ball, I held my shoulder with my other hand, expecting him to feel sorry for the pain he had caused. Instead of an apology, he grabbed his own shoulder and with a sneer and some sarcasm, made mocking, crying noises like a baby with diaper rash. Realizing that the opposition only rejoiced in my injury and that he would hit me again if given the chance was intimidating and discouraging. But then I looked at my teammates. They were concerned. They cared. Additionally, my teammates were counting on me. If I chose to hide behind my injury and use it as an excuse to quit trying, I would let them down and we would all lose. The only thing I could do was buckle down and play with an injured shoulder for the rest of the tournament.

　　从这仿佛一记重击的经验里，我学到一个宝贵的教训：就算我终身处于"精神受伤"的状态，这个世界也不会停止旋转，和我竞争的人更不会因此手下留情。如果我选择和我的疾病妥协，而放弃追求生活中的"胜利"，那么与我对立的病魔会轻松获胜，并当着我的面大肆嘲笑我。一味同情自己、用疾病作为借口，而放弃名为"人生"的这场比赛，是一个注定失败的主意。那不仅会让我自己变得无用，也让关心我的人同样尝到失败的滋味。不！绝对不要这么做。拒绝作战与躲在借口后面都不是正确的方式，掌握、控制好我的疾病，并持续前进才是正确的方法。然而我该如何采取不同的行动来控制好我的疾病呢？我一直思索该如何在"精神受伤"的状态中继续这场人生游戏，最后我发觉，有一件事情我可以轻松掌握，那就是吃药的时间点。

From that school of hard knocks experience, I learned the world wouldn't unwind and the competition wouldn't give in simply because I had a permanent "mental injury." If I chose to give in to the tendencies of my illness and quit striving for life's victories, the opposition would win and laugh in my face about it. Feeling sorry for myself and using my disorder as an excuse to quit playing the game of life was a lose-lose deal. It not only crippled me personally, it also forfeited the win for those who cared for me. No. Stopping the fight and hiding behind excuses was not the answer. Taking control and pressing forward was. But what could I do differently to take control? As I thought about how I could stay in the game of life while playing with a "mental injury," I found one simple thing I could control was the time I took my medications.

　　与其在睡前把当天的药量一次吃进去，我改成在早上当抑郁症最严重的时候吃抗抑郁的药，而把抗躁药改在晚上我需要安静的时候再吃。花了好几个星期，我的身体才习惯这个用药模式，但一段时间后效果就慢慢出来了。我仍然比一般人晚起床而且也上床晚，但在我清醒的期间里情绪确实比较稳定。在这段控制吃药时间的过程中，我开始能注意到我的身体情况，以及会对我身体产生不同影响的事物。我发觉晚上打篮球直到午夜，会让躁狂症状增强，使我完全不能睡觉，从此我就提早运动，好让晚上身体依然会劳累，但头脑不致太有精神。这样运动不只让我睡得比较好，同时也降低了白天的抑郁程度。我还发现食物也会影响躁狂和抑郁的症状，睡觉前喝含咖啡因的饮料以及吃甜点，对我情绪的影响犹如在夜间打球。

　　Instead of taking all my pills right before bed, I took my antidepressants in the morning when depression hit hardest and my antipsychotic meds at night when I needed to settle down. It took several weeks for my body to get used to the change, but over time it started working. I still slept in later than most and I still went to bed later than most, but I became more stable during the hours I was awake. During this process of controlling when I took my medicine, I became more aware of my body and the different influences on it. I started noticing that playing basketball until midnight enhanced mania and made it impossible to sleep. I started exercising earlier so I would be tired physically, but not worked up mentally at bedtime. The exercise not only helped me to sleep better, it also lessened my depression during the day. I also noticed that my diet influenced mania and depression. Caffeine drinks and sugar treats before bed had the same effect as late night basketball.

于是我开始注意饮食，吃健康的食物，这样做不仅减轻白天的抑郁程度，并且帮助我控制夜晚时的躁狂程度。控制我的吃药时间、运动及饮食，让我有办法驾驭大脑。然而当我注意到它的需求，尽力开往一条比以前稳定的生活道路时，又碰上一个新问题；改变吃药和生活方式，让我得以驾驭自己思想油门的速度和强弱，不过我的头脑还是有毛病。当这部"赛车"跑不动的时候，我立刻发觉我必须要检查"燃料"的存量，换句话说，我必须要学习如何控制思想的"内容"。于是我决定雇请专业的"维修团队"给我提供咨询。我的心理顾问帮助我开始把健康的自我期许和务实的目标这类"燃料""加"到我的思想里，她也教导我"认为自己应该要如何如何"的想法，是会污染我的思想的。

I started watching my diet and ate more healthy foods. These changes also dampened my depression during the day and helped to manage my mania at night. Taking control of my meds, my physical activity, and my diet put me in my brain's driver seat. However, as I listened to its needs and tried to steer toward a more stable life, I found a new problem. The pills and lifestyle changes helped control the speed and intensity of my racing thoughts, but often my brain still sputtered, coughed, and wheezed. I soon realized that I needed to check the "fuel" inside. In other words, I needed to learn how to control the *content* of my thoughts. That's when I decided to hire a "pit crew" and get professional counseling. My counselor helped me to start fueling my thoughts with healthy self-expectations and realistic goals. She taught me how showering myself with "shoulds" polluted my mind.

例如"我应该是最棒的""我应该更努力工作，这样我生活中的一切就会完美"，或者"我应该时时感到快乐"……诸如此类的想法，就像是脏污的油灌进我的思想，因为那些想法是永远无法达成的。我的心理顾问教我用鼓励性的想法来代替，例如"我尽力而为了""我工作很努力，所以现在可以休息""有时候不开心也没有什么关系"等等，用这些积极、正面的想法来清除我那有问题的"完美主义"。我的顾问还告诉我有许多其他的"精神燃料"，可以帮助我脑中的引擎得以发动得更顺畅。由于音乐对我的影响力非常大，所以我对音乐的选择变得非常谨慎。其中我所找到对我的精神最有助益的"燃料"之一，就是只听那些使我感到快乐而且歌词振奋人心的歌，摒弃或远离那些播放负面或沮丧音乐的 CD 片或电台。

Statements like "I should be the best. " "If I don't always get what I want it's because I didn't work hard enough. " or, "I should be happy all the time. " were like dumping dirty oil into my mind because they were impossible to achieve. My counselor also taught me that empowering thoughts like "I am doing my best. " "I worked hard. It's okay to rest now. " Or, "It is okay not to feel happy all the time. " cleansed my mind with positive reality and washed out the impurities of perfectionism. My counselor taught me about many other "mental fuels" that helped my mind's engine to run more smoothly. Since music had such a powerful influence on me, I became very cautious about the songs I listened to. Ditching the depressing, downer CDs and radio stations while searching out and soothing my soul with uplifting and inspiring music became one of my greatest sources of excellent emotional fuel.

　　稳坐在"驾驶"座上，让干净、健康的"燃料"充满我心中的燃料箱，确实帮助我控制住了奔驰的心。然而在赛道上奔驰，只是没有目标的不断绕圈子。虽然我开始能掌控我自己，但我在生活上其实没什么方向。我起床，开车去上课，开车回家，开车去上班，开车回家，然后上床睡觉。隔天醒来，我还是做同样的事。我总是在怀疑为什么我只是在原地打转？有时候我甚至不知道自己究竟是醒着还是在做梦，因为我过的生活就好像一场噩梦；也许你做过这样的噩梦——不管喝了多少饮料、吃了多少东西，仍然觉得又渴又饿？事实上，我最常做的噩梦是我想要不断地跑厕所。在梦中，虽然我一次又一次去上厕所，但总感觉还是需要再去一趟。不管是哪一种噩梦，唯一能从饥饿——或是下腹亟须解放的压力中——解脱的方式就是醒过来。

Sitting in the driver's seat and filling up my own gas tank with clean and healthy "fuel" helped me take control of my racing mind. However, driving on a racetrack only meant going in circles. Although I was in control, my life wasn't really going anywhere. I woke up. I drove to school. I drove home. I drove to work. I drove home. I went to bed. The next day I did the same thing. Round and round I went, all the while wondering why I wasn't going anywhere. Sometimes I didn't know if I was awake or asleep. My life was passing like a bad dream. You know the one…no matter how much you eat or drink, you still feel hungry and thirsty? Actually the dream I have most often is the one where I have to use the restroom. In that dream I go to the bathroom over and over again, but I still have to go. Whatever the dream, the only way to satisfy the hunger – or the pressing need for relief – is to wake up.

　　"大觉醒"止是我所需要的，能让我停止绕圈子，并且开始向更值得前往的方向前进。所以，你是不是想问我是如何醒过来的？在那饥饿的梦中，你是否感觉到对食物迫切的需求？你是不是一直在吞吃着手边所及的一切，但仍饥渴地寻找真正能填饱你的东西？秘密就在这儿：当你仔细看最棒、最有用的生命之料理时，你会发现"永恒恩爱关系"是那能解除饥渴的水、让生命一直"吃饱"的白饭，以及所有能滋养灵魂的料理中最重要的材料。生命是一片你置身其中的汪洋，心理疾病是当你在海面击水挣扎时，掀起滔天大浪的强风；药物和精神病专家是搭救你的救护艇，你渴望找回永恒恩爱的关系则是给你控制力及目的的舵，让你可以朝着正确的方向前进。

　　A "great awakening" was exactly what I needed to do to stop driving in circles and start driving toward a worthwhile destination. So how did I "wake up" you ask? Do you feel a pressing need? Are you eating and eating, but still starving for an answer? Here is the secret. Look in life's greatest and most proven cookbook and you'll see "eternal, loving relationships" are the water that quenches, the rice that fills, and the other most basic ingredients for all soul-nourishing recipes. Life is an ocean you have fallen into. Mental illness is a wind that blows mountainous waves over you as you try to tread water. The pills and professionals are a life-saving boat you climb into. Your desire to return to eternal loving relationships is the rudder that gives you the control and purpose you need to steer a straight course.

　　我相信没有被察觉、不愿被承认、不被明白，或没有被好好控制的心理疾病会让你感到孤独，觉得自己像在漫无目的的躁狂飓风和抑郁低潮以及其他难受的症状之间，不断被冲来漂去；但千万不要被误导，以为你会因这个疾病而再也不能在人生中拥有那些甜美的关系。

　　真正的美好风景正等着你：当你一旦踏上"控制"这块踏脚石时，你会看见、听见那些真诚的朋友们和关心你的家人们——他们正不断地为你加油，鼓励你走向那在远处的宁静水流，他们正在那里等着迎接并给你热情的拥抱——你只是因为疾病造成的混乱而从未知道，他们其实一直都在那里。

I believe unidentified, unauthorized, misunderstood, and uncontrolled mental illness can make you feel all alone, drifting aimlessly amid hurricanes and doldrums of mania, depression, and other terrible symptoms. Don't be misled into thinking that because you have mental illness you can't have loving relationships again in your life. The beauty of reaching the stepping-stone "Control" is that once you are there, you will be able to see and hear the many true friends and caring family members cheering you on toward the distant, calm waters where they wait to greet and embrace you. They have always been there; you just never realized it because of the fury of the illness around you.

借着相信能找回永恒恩爱关系、专业的辅导、定时定期服用医生开的药物、有计划的运动及健康的饮食，我控制了我的疾病，让我的生活得以再度找回平衡。现在，我不再甘于过着只求生存的人生了，我渴望能提升我的生活，让我不只是远远地看着亲友们，而是能脱离心理疾病的激流，和他们一起在正常的水流里生活。因此，"提升"就是我需要达到的最后一块踏脚石。

By believing I could find eternal, loving relationships, and through professional counseling, scheduled prescription medications, planned exercise, and eating a healthy diet, I took control of my illness and brought balance back into my life. Now, I wouldn't settle for simply surviving. I wanted a *heightened* life where I could not just see my family and friends in the distance, but I could join them in the manageable "normal" waters away from the mental illness rapids. "Heighten," turned out to be the last stepping-stone I needed in order to reach them.

第六章 步骤五：提升你的生活方式

爱就是幸福

活着就是爱

我曾从电视上看到一则让我很感动的广告：广告一开始，一个年轻的小男孩把一台摄影机装进防水的夹链袋。那个孩子可爱、天真、神情专注，让我不禁露出微笑，不知道他到底想做什么？接着，他把装着摄影机的夹链袋封紧，把它放到洗碗机里面，关上洗碗机的门，然后按下"开始清洗"的按钮。在广告的最后一幕，当小男孩看着他所"制作"的影片大笑时，画面上出现了一行标语："保留好奇心"。我很喜欢那句话，因为它给了我所需要的鼓励。虽然我的躁郁症已经被察觉、承认、明白，而且控制得宜，但我发现自己仍会慢慢地滑进抑郁或躁狂所引起的忧闷状态里。

Chapter 6
Step Five: Heighten Your Life

Love is happiness

Living is loving

I once saw an inspiring commercial for public TV. It began with a young child stuffing a video recorder into a clear, water tight zip-lock bag. The cute, innocent, and determined look on his face made me smile. I wondered what his intentions were. After zipping the bag shut, he stuck the package into the dishwasher, closed the door, and pressed the "wash" button. In the final scene, as the young boy laughed at the picture he produced, the slogan, "Stay Curious" flew onto the screen. I loved the message because it gave me encouragement that I needed to hear. Even though my bipolar disorder was identified, authorized, understood, and controlled, I found myself slowly slipping into a depressed or manic "blah" mode.

　　处在忧闷状态中，就像是高速公路旁虽然绽放了数百朵野生的向日葵，但当我开车经过时，却完全不会注意到这些美丽的花朵。在这种状态时的我，会在热闹的派对中呵欠连连、边跳舞边做白日梦，还有在日出的美景前打盹。你可以想象我在这种情况下和人聊天是什么样子吧——不知所云、不着边际而且非常无聊。相对地，在躁狂引起的烦闷状态中，则像是在夜里出现可怕的闪电霹雳、雷声隆隆，还有不停的暴雨，但我却专注在自己的工作里，而没有注意到外界的变化。这种状态会导致我行事不经思考、过于情绪化，甚至送出具有攻击性的言辞和邮件，让我在别人不同意或误解我的想法时，用很不谨慎，或气势汹汹的方式沟通。在这些忧闷状态中，我会疏于防卫我的疾病，于是我的病开始偷走我对生活的好奇心、我体贴别人的能力，以及我对生命的热爱。任由这些事情从我身上被夺走，就是允许我的对手（心理疾病）获得更多优势。

In depressed "blah" mode hundreds of wild sunflowers bloomed along the highway, but I drooped by without noticing. Depressed "blah" mode made me yawn at parties, daydream at dances, and snooze through sunrises. You can guess what conversations started to sound like while I was in this mode… "blah, blah, blah." In manic "blah" mode, flashing lightning, pulsing thunder, and streaking raindrops filled the nighttime air with thrilling electricity…but I worked right through it. Manic "blah" mode resulted in not-thought-out, over-emotional, and even offensive letters and emails. Manic "blah" mode made me speak carelessly with overbearing force when someone disagreed with or misunderstood me. In "blah" mode I let down my guard. Consequently, my illness started to steal away my curiosity, my concern for others, and my love of life. Allowing these elements to be taken from me allowed my mental illness enemy to gain the advantage.

　　在我的人生走到这个阶段之前，我一直把我的心理疾病视为必须征服的敌人，我的一天总是从能否起床的自我战争中展开，接着是为了在一整天中都保持清醒而战斗。每个晚上，为了让自己能放松睡着，我同样必须持续和疾病对抗。在前述的郁闷状态中，要打赢在我脑袋里的化学战争是不可能的。然而，那则电视广告不只是激励我逃脱这个心理状态，并找到方法保持对生活的好奇心，它同时也给了我灵感，让我用另一种眼光来面对心理疾病。我想到广告里的小男孩，他是如何把一个挑战视为一个让他感到喜悦的机会，于是在我心里产生了这样的想法："也许要战胜这郁闷状态的秘密，只是单纯地停止我每天的'躁郁战争'？""与其和躁郁症一味地对抗，或许我可以和它们和平共处，一起共同创造出一些好东西出来？"

　　Up until that point in my life, I had always viewed my mental illness as an enemy to be conquered. My days began with a battle to wake up in the morning. Then, I fought to stay awake all day. Every night the strife continued as I struggled to go to sleep. In "blah" mode, it was impossible to win the chemical war in my head. The TV commercial not only motivated me to get out of "blah" mode and find a way to "stay curious" in life, it also inspired a change in the way I viewed my mental illness. Thinking about how the young boy used a challenge as an opportunity to experience joy, the thought came to me, "Maybe the secret of conquering 'blah' mode is to simply quit fighting these 'bipolar battles' all the time." I thought, "Maybe instead of combating them, I can make peace and use my mania and depression as allies to create something good."

　　这是一个关键的时刻：我决定停止对疾病的作战，并开始运用它来提升我的生活。那天夜里，我不再躺在床上强迫自己入眠，反而起身写一首钓鱼的诗。因为当时我正处在躁郁症中躁狂的那一端，所以情绪高昂、充满创造力，且有源源不绝的灵感。我知道这些感觉来自于躁狂症，而且隔天早上起来时，就不会再觉得我所写的诗有多高明，不过我的态度是："我可以享受当下的感觉，不用去在乎明天是否期望落空。"到了睡意出现时，我不勉强自己熬夜来享受躁狂症带来的过瘾感受，而是心满意足地爬上床，并且很快就睡着了。在闭上眼睛睡觉之前，我看了看闹钟，发现跟我通常能入睡的时间其实是一样的。用写诗取代躺在床上失眠好几个小时，是我利用晚上的躁狂症为自己带来益处的第一个方法。几年以后，我写的诗足以让我出版一本叫作《鳟鱼学院：豪钓者渔歌》（A School of Trout：A Spirited Stringer of Fishing Poetry）的诗集。

This was the point when I decided to stop warring my illness, and start using it to heighten my life. That night, instead of lying in bed fighting desperately to force myself to sleep, I got up and started writing a poem about fishing. Being on the manic side of the bipolar cycle, I felt motivated, creative, and inspired. I understood it was just mania, and that in the morning the poem wouldn't seem as ingenious, but I figured, "I'll enjoy the feeling for now, and not hold high expectations tomorrow." When I started feeling tired, instead of fighting to stay up and keep enjoying the mania, I climbed into bed and went right to sleep. Before dosing off, I glanced at the clock and realized it was the same time I always fell asleep. Writing fishing poetry instead of lying in bed for hours was the first way I started using nighttime mania to my advantage. Eventually, I composed enough poetry to publish a book titled, "A School of Trout：A Spirited Stringer of Fishing Poetry."

　　我原以为，就像别人无法体会我在躁狂症之下所感到的兴奋一样，他们也不会觉得我的诗有任何令人惊喜之处。但这个想法大错特错了！全美国甚至加拿大都有人购买我的书，有些卖飞标钓鱼零售店的老板询问我，可不可以在他们的文宣品、网站、钓鱼用品上印上我的诗；有位报社记者写信问我，能不能在她某篇有关钓鱼的文章里引用我的一首诗。还有一本名为《Fishing Wyoming》的杂志开了"钓鱼诗人专栏"，用近一年的时间每个月刊登一首不同的诗。"9·11事件"后一星期，在一个广播节目中，那位DJ表示他感到那天在节目中分享的钓鱼诗让节目的气氛适当且感动人心——即使这是个以野外为主题的节目。朋友在他们的演讲上引用我的作品，我还收到一封邮件，是一位女士询问是否能在她刚过世的亲爱父亲的葬礼悼文中引用我的诗作。

　　I figured that just like others didn't feel the same enthusiasm I did when I was manic, people would not think my poetry was anything to get excited about. However, like trout on a chain, I was dead wrong. People from all over the United States and even Canada bought the book. Some asked if they could use poems in the book for their fly shop newsletters, websites, and fishing products. A newspaper columnist asked to use one of the poems in her article on fishing. "Fishing Wyoming" magazine made a feature called "Fish Poets' Corner" and published a different poem each month for several months. During a radio interview one week following the 9/11 attacks, the DJ commented that the fishing poetry we read on the air created an appropriate and thoughtful mood - even for an outdoors show. Religious friends shared my fishing poems in their speeches. I even received an email request to use a poem from my book in a eulogy for a beloved father.

　　写作并出版一本书是我一次梦想成真的经验。由于每天只专注于跟我的心理疾病作战，我好像虚度了好多年，完全没有把自己的梦想放在心上。与我的病和平相处，终于使战争的烟雾散去，此后我才开始看到在我身边的诸多可能性，并再次相信梦想。而当我再度打开心扉、相信梦想时，许多使梦想成真的机会，就像是饥饿的鳟鱼向美味的蜉蝣奔泳而来一样不断地出现。我唯一需要做的，就是从我脑中的"逐梦钓具箱"里，找出合适的鱼钩来。我抛出的第一个钓梦之"钩"，完美地符合了这些"机会之鱼"的胃口。在我出版了那本钓鱼诗集后不久，2002 年盐湖城冬季奥运会开始筹办，寻找义工。当我听到他们的广告，我知道我会说中文的能力会是那正确的"鱼钩"，让我可以把握住这个千载难逢的机会，我的心因此充满了勇气。

Writing and publishing a book was a dream come true. Focusing on my daily battles with my mental illness had allowed years to pass since I had even thought about any personal dreams. Making peace with my illness allowed the smoke of battle to clear. Only then did I start to see the possibilities around me and to again believe in dreams. As I began to open my mind to dreams again, opportunities to live them started rising like hungry trout in a mayfly hatch. All I needed to do was search in my mind's "dream-holder tackle box" and find the right hook. One of the first "dream hooks" I dug up matched the hatch of opportunity perfectly. Not long after publishing my poetry book, a call went out for volunteers to help make the 2002 winter Olympics in Salt Lake City the best games ever. When I heard the advertisement and realized my Chinese language ability could be the right "hook" to catch this once in a lifetime opportunity, my mind and heart took courage.

　　我递出申请书之后不久，我的战利品马上就上钩了，我于是很快地收线，捕获我的奥运梦想。经过好几个月的训练，终于收到了特派给我的奥运任务。我打开任务信封时手一直在发抖，接下来读到内文让我的心沸腾——我获选为国际奥运会（IOC）中国台湾代表吴经国博士的专任助理！当吴博士的司机并协助他和他的家人，真是梦想成真的经验。站在他身边，我得以结识几位奥运的大明星，例如 Carl Lewis（卡尔·刘易斯，美籍短跑名人）、Kristi Yamaguchi（山口克丽丝蒂，日裔美籍溜冰名人），还与一些知名的美国社会与政府领导人擦身而过，如国防部长 Donald Rumsfeld，犹他州州长 Mike Leavitt，NBA 犹他州爵士队的大老板 Larry Miller，还有将要入美式橄榄球 NFL 名人堂（Hall of Fame）的 Steve Young。

When I cast out my application, a trophy catch immediately struck and I began reeling in my Olympic dream. After months of training, I finally received my specific Olympic assignment. My hands shook as I opened the envelope. What I read caused my heart to soar. I had been selected to be the dedicated assistant for Dr. Ching Kuo Wu, the IOC (International Olympic Committee) representative from Chinese Taiwan! Driving and assisting Dr. Wu and his family turned into a dream come true. Standing by his side, I got to meet and mingle with Olympic stars like Carl Lewis, and Kristi Yamaguchi. I got to rub shoulders with prominent community and government leaders like Secretary of Defense, Donald Rumsfeld, Governor Mike Leavitt, Utah Jazz owner, Larry Miller, and future NFL Hall of Famer, Steve Young.

　　吴先生邀请我在门票早已被卖光的贵宾席上和他一起坐，我也有荣幸认识且一起跟中国大陆（何振梁先生与夫人）和泰国参与国际奥运会的委员们吃年夜饭。在吴先生要帮忙颁奖时，我有机会跟他一起到后台，当时我差点要捏自己看是否在梦里！这个奥运梦里最好的部分，就是跟吴博士的家庭成为朋友。在他们返回中国台湾之前，吴先生和他的妻子到我的家里来，认识了我的太太跟小孩。我们一起坐在饭桌前用毛笔画水墨画、写书法，那幅吴氏夫妇签名的艺术品，现在还放在我的办公室里。它常提醒我：梦想可以成真——即使是心理疾病的病患也行。有句中国成语说"水往低处流，人往高处走。"因为心理疾病的原因，长期以来我并不相信这话对我而言也是有意义的。

　　Mr. Wu invited me to sit with him in the front row, VIP seating at sold out events. I had the honor of meeting and sharing a Chinese New Year feast with IOC members from China （Mr. Zhen Liang He and his wife） and Thailand. I even got to go back stage when Mr. Wu participated in a medal presentation. I had to pinch myself often to believe the dream was real! The best part of living my Olympic dream was becoming friends with the Wu family. Before they left for home, Dr. Wu and his wife came to my house to meet my wife and children. Together we sat at the kitchen table and made Chinese art pieces. The piece he and his wife signed sits in my office to this day. It is a constant reminder to me that dreams can come true – even to those with mental illness. An ancient Chinese idiom says, "Water rolls down, but man climbs up the mountain." For too long I believed this saying didn't apply to me because I had mental illness.

但在这场冬季奥运的美好经验之后，我不再让自己像水一般一直往下跌，而开始像个真正的男人一样往上爬。爬上更高层次生活的关键秘诀，就是看见、相信，并一直朝着梦想往前进。很多很多患心理疾病的人认为他们的梦想已经永远被夺去，也许你是其中一位。我希望在这里告诉你，心理疾病并不会夺走梦想，只会把它从你眼前藏起来。再次把梦想找出来的秘诀就是继续"往前走"，直到你走出脑海里遮住视野的"雾"为止。你知道你的梦想是什么，这梦想就在你的心里，把它们发掘出来，把握它们，并朝着它们努力使它们成真，即使你以为自己完全看不到它们。这就是我需要去寻找并且发现的最大梦想。其实，在我还没听过"躁郁症"这种东西之前，我生平最大的渴望，就是娶到我的梦中佳人，并和她一起组织家庭。

After the Olympics, I stopped dripping downward like water, and started hiking upward like a man. The secret to climbing to a "heightened" life was seeing, believing in, and pressing forward toward dreams. There are many, many people with mental illness who feel their dreams have been stolen away forever. Maybe you are one of them. I'm here to tell you mental illness doesn't steal away dreams. It only hides them from your view. The secret to rediscovering your dreams is to continue "pressing forward" until you find your way out of the fog. You know your dreams. They are there inside your heart. Dig them up, hold on to them, and work toward them, even if you feel like you can't see them anymore. This is what I had to do to find and realize my greatest dream. Even before I had ever heard of bipolar disorder, my life's greatest desire was to marry the girl of my dreams and raise a family together.

我一直紧抓着这个最大的梦想，即使来自躁郁症的猛烈冲击使我受伤、盲目而一度看不见我的梦，即使感觉快要迷失自我，我的梦想就像一根安全的铁杆，让我能用所有的力气和意志紧握着它，并陪着我在这许多年通过黑暗、沮丧的幽雾往前走，最终带领我的梦抵达光明的一端。现在，我当然知道结婚生子并不是对每个躁郁症或其他任何心理疾病的病患都适用的答案，这不是我想强调的重点；重点是你要知道什么是你的梦想，不要让心理疾病卷起的乌云左右你，让你误以为你的梦想已经消失。你的梦想始终存在，如果你一直坚持朝着它前进，最终必定会拨云见日，实现你的梦想。当你思考你心中的梦想的时候，很重要的一点是：要记住幻想与现实之间的区别。通常当我们思及梦想的时候，总会联想到明亮灿烂的日落光辉，以及美好如置身天堂的幸福世界。

I held on to this "greatest" dream even when bipolar disorder socked me so hard that I became blind to dreams. Even though it felt like I had become lost, my dream became an iron safety handrail that I held onto with all my strength and determination. Pressing forward through the years of dark and depressed fog, the safety handrail eventually led me onward until the dream came into the light. Now, I know that marriage and children aren't the answer for everyone suffering from bipolar disorder or any other mental illness. That's not the point. The point is that you know your dream. Don't let the clouds of mental illness make you believe your dream is gone. The dream is still there and if you constantly press forward toward it, eventually the clouds will clear. As you think of your dreams, it's important to remember the difference between fantasy and reality. Often, when we think of dreams, we think of bright, setting sunrays and perfect heavenly bliss.

　　我们看过那么多"从此过着幸福快乐日子"的电影，所以我们开始以为新生活也将会像这样。其实当我生活中最大的梦想实现时，我仍然跟自己的疾病在苦斗，即使我活在最大的梦想里：结了婚有了孩子，我依旧受苦于躁郁症的纠缠。即使现在，我也不能说我的生活就跟西部电影里牛仔策马走向落日的经典情节一样潇洒完美；日落后一定会天黑，若想让梦想不随着夕阳沉没，势必得付出努力与牺牲。婚姻并不容易——连没有躁郁症的人也不得不同意这一点。大声哭闹的婴儿，就可以让没有心理疾病的人体验到濒临崩溃的感受。有时躁郁的黑雾一样会盖住梦想的乐观光辉，但困难并未使我放弃，我不断地尽全力前进，因为我知道，我的梦想就是那条引导我抵达长久快乐的道路。

　　We see so many movies where they live "happily ever after" that we start to believe life is that way. This isn't reality. Reaching my life's greatest dream actually happened while I was still battling my disorder. Even while I was married with children and "living my life's greatest dream." I still suffered bouts with manic breakdowns and extreme depression. Even now, I can't say I'm "riding off into the sunset." The sun that sets *will* be followed by darkness. That is the time when keeping the dream alive takes work and sacrifice. Marriage is tough – even for people who don't have bipolar disorder. Screaming babies can bring a feeling of insanity even to people who aren't mentally ill. Sometimes clouds of darkness cover the "silver lining" of my dream. But that doesn't mean I quit. I am determined to continue to press forward, because I know my dream is actually my road to lasting happiness.

　　你怎么知道你所选的路会使你通往快乐呢？答案就是：当你的梦想一个一个以彼此为基础不断建立起来的同时，你的生活也会随之不断提升的话，你就可以知道这条路是对的了。比如说，我哄儿子睡觉的时候，我希望再度唱歌的梦也实现了。当我渴望听到我女儿的笑声时，她和我一起跳舞，舞步便驱散了那些盖住我的跳舞梦想的黑雾。在我想取悦我妻子时，我也同时建造了梦想的家园。所有这些梦想，都是一步跟着一步建立起来的，我的生活也一点一点随之提升。当我在这条快乐道路上不断前进时，美丽的梦想也像春季的黄水仙般，不断地在我身边开放。有时候我确实可以感觉到有温暖喜乐的阳光，其他的时候我则必须用扯破的雨伞忍受名为躁郁的暴风雨。不论我能否感受到这一切，我知道自己正在过一种不断向上提升的生活。

　　How do you know when you have chosen the road toward your happiness? The answer is that you know you are on the road to happiness when dreams build on each other and your life continues to heighten. For example, while helping my son go to sleep, my dream of singing again came true. Wanting to hear my daughter laugh, she and I waltzed away the clouds that had covered my dream of dancing again. Hoping to please my wife, I found myself digging the home of our dreams out of the dirt. All these dreams built on themselves and each lifted my life a little bit higher. By simply pressing forward on my road of happiness, dreams continue to bloom around me like daffodils in springtime. Sometimes I can feel the rays of joyful sunlight. Other times I have to put up my tattered umbrella and endure the blinding and deafening storms. Whether I can feel it or not, I know I am living a "heightened" life.

毕竟，快乐的定义不就是"奋起并成就梦想"吗？当与爱我的亲友站在比较平静的生活水流中，回顾已越过的心理疾病急流时，我知道这疾病其实是个祝福。首先，为了发现并爬上那巨大的"谦卑之石"，我得学习如何接受教导且愿意改善自己。找到第一个踏脚石并察觉我的疾病，让我学习究竟什么是精神病，更帮我克服自己的傲慢无知。能够看透（心理疾病的）表面症状之后，使我了解母亲与其他精神病人的痛苦——他们并不是自找麻烦的疯子；相反地，他们是不同寻常的人，只是得了一种跟中风或小儿麻痹类似的疾病而已。"察觉"自身的疾病，帮助我踏出前往平静水流的下一步。在那一块踏脚石上我学习到的是：自己有弱点并没有关系。

After all, isn't the definition of happiness, "rising up and living our greatest dreams?" As I stand in more stable and peaceful waters, surrounded by loving family and friends, I can now look back on the mental illness rapids I have navigated. I can see that the disorder is actually a blessing. First, by finding and climbing the great boulder "humility," I became teachable and willing to change myself for the better. Finding the first stepping – stone and *identifying* my illness helped educate me about mental illness and allowed me to overcome my arrogant ignorance. Learning to see past "surface symptoms" helped me to understand my own mother and others with mental illness. They weren't crazies who brought their plight upon themselves. They were exceptional people with a disorder just like a stroke or polio. *Authorizing* illness in myself helped me take the next step toward peaceful waters. On that stepping—stone I learned it was okay to have weakness.

拥有弱点能打开我的眼睛和心扉，让我接纳那些倚靠药物过生活的人，也教导我在真正需要帮助的时候请求他人的协助并不丢脸。"承认"我的疾病则让我在别人的眼里是个普通人；承认我有心理疾病，不会叫他人觉得我是弱者，反而证明我有坚强的力量面对疾病。"明白"真正的自己与疾病两者的差异，让我从过去躁郁症所带来的纠结中获得释放，使我了解隐藏在我脑海的可怕思想以及沉闷抑郁只是病状而非真正的我——我只是一个生了病的好人。

从"明白"跳往下一个踏脚石的时候，我看到脚下清澈的水中映着自己的倒影，却也看见心理疾病的影子永远与我形影不离，让我差点失去"控制"。

It opened my eyes and heart to others who relied upon medications. It taught me to stop being ashamed of asking for help when I needed it. Authorizing my illness made me seem like a real person to others. Instead of giving the impression of a weakling, admitting I had a mental illness actually demonstrated strength. *Understanding* the difference between me and my illness was a stepping-stone that allowed me to break free from the tangled knots and manic highs of my past. It was comforting to understand that the scary thoughts and demented depression I repressed deep in my mind were only an illness and they were *not* me. I was a good person with a shadowy disorder. As I jumped from "Understand" toward the next stepping-stone, I glanced down into the clear water and saw my own reflection. Seeing the mental illness shadow permanently attached to me almost made me lose *control*.

为了让自己恢复平衡，我开始在固定的时间用药，改变运动的作息，吃健康食物。给我生活最大的方向感和意义的就是再次相信并追求恒久恩爱的关系。相信梦想可以成真，让我从"控制"跳上最后一块踏脚石："提升"。在那儿我得到了朋友与家人关爱的拥抱，他们一直在那里替我加油，并且为我祈祷，祈求神让我能安全逃离危险的躁郁症急流。虽然现在的我并没有得到完全的医治，但是我生活的水流的确比以前平缓了许多。于是，我渴望伸出手来，帮助那些还在躁郁症水流中摇荡的人。我心中满怀祈祷和爱，衷心地把这本书当作装了援助资讯的瓶中信送进水流。抓牢它，研读它！说不定这五块踏脚石，正是帮你通过心理疾病急流而达到平静生活的援助。

In order to catch my balance, I started scheduling the time of day or night I took my meds. I changed my exercise schedule and started eating healthy foods. Believing in eternal, loving relationships gave me the power I need to gain direction and meaning in my life again. Believing in dreams helped me skip from "Control" to the last stepping-stone, "Heighten." There I reached and embraced the arms of loving friends and family. They had always been there, cheering and praying for my safe deliverance out of the treacherous rapids. So here I am today. Not completely cured, but wading in waters that are much more stable and peaceful. Now that I'm here, I want to offer my helping hand to those still swirling and tumbling in rough waters. With a prayer in my heart and in the spirit of love, I'm sending out this book as a message in a bottle. Grab it! Study it. Maybe these five stepping-stones are just the help you need to navigate the rapids of your mental illness and allow you to reach a more peaceful life.

自助手册

以下的"自助手册"分为两部分：第一部分是专为患了躁郁症的人而写的，第二部分则是给他们的照顾者、家人与友人；欢迎大家两个部分都看，两者都是要指引你运用书里的五个步骤，得到更平静的生活。使用这些步骤时，要像使用牢靠的手杖来涉过脚底下有滑溜石头的急流一样，每一步都要很谨慎；要思考，要小心。不要急躁，不要试图跳过任何步骤。当你研读并操作时，请利用你自己的日记或其他笔记本写下笔记和心得。写这样的日记就像是在最烈的日光底下给你戴的太阳眼镜。它可以帮你更深入、更详尽地检视心中的感受，更清楚地看到你的思想和动机，而且能帮助你回顾并发现自己的进步与成长。

Self-Help Workbook

This self-help "workshop" is in two parts. The first is written specifically for people with bipolar disorder. The second is for their caregivers, family and friends. Feel free to read both. Each is a guide to lead you through the five steps toward a more peaceful life. They are written to be a hands-on reference to be used like you would a sturdy walking stick while wading on slippery rocks through a raging river. Take each step carefully, thoughtfully, and seriously. Don't rush. Don't try to skip ahead. As you read and work, use the space provided at the end of each step to keep notes and to write your thoughts. Keeping a journal is like a pair of prescription sunglasses in the bright sun. They help you to view your feelings with deeper detail, to see your thoughts and motivations more clearly, and they allow you to look back and notice progress and improvement.

　　在你学习并依靠这本"手杖"与"太阳眼镜"时，千万不要忘记你要前往的目的地。你可以做得到！躁郁症是可以治疗的，更平静的水流是能够抵达的。

As you lean on your walking stick and look through your enlightening shades, never forget the destination you are working toward. You can make it! Bipolar disorder is treatable. More peaceful waters are obtainable.

第七章　写给躁郁症病患

先决条件：征服谦卑之石

在你要踏上通过五块踏脚石的旅程之前，换句话说，在你接受我或任何其他人的帮助之前，你必须要先通过"谦卑之石"的考验。征服谦卑之石的方法，就是学会并表现"我需要帮助""我有弱点""我愿意听取别人建议来改变我自己"的态度。

为什么在走向更平静生活的旅途时，使自己谦卑是那么必要呢？有几个原因，请你思考一下：

Chapter 7
For Those With Bipolar Disorder

Prerequisite：CONQUER ROCK HUMILITY

Before you can start on the five-step journey, or in other words, before you will ever accept the help I, or anyone else offers, you must first "conquer rock humility." The way to "conquer rock humility" is to grasp and accept the attitude of, "I need help. I have weakness. I am willing to listen to others and change myself." Why is humility so necessary to start on the journey toward a more peaceful life? Here are some reasons to think about：

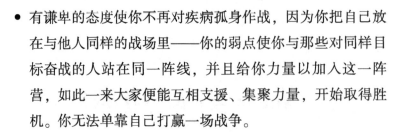

- 有谦卑的态度使你不再对疾病孤身作战，因为你把自己放在与他人同样的战场里——你的弱点使你与那些对同样目标奋战的人站在同一阵线，并且给你力量以加入这一阵营，如此一来大家便能互相支援、集聚力量，开始取得胜机。你无法单靠自己打赢一场战争。

- 有谦卑的态度使你开始察觉身边的人要提供给你的大力帮助，也会因获得旁人更多关心而感到轻松和被支持，因为你会停止批评他们不完美的地方，而且停止假装自己不需要改变。

- 有谦卑的态度使你的困惑转变成明白，因为你会从许多人的心智中得到教导，而不再企图依赖染病的心理来寻找解答。

- With humility you stop fighting your illness alone because you put yourself on the same battlefield as others who also are warring "your weakness." Putting yourself on the same level with them allows you to draw on their combined strength, and gives you the power to join forces and start winning battles you couldn't win alone.

- With humility you start to recognize the generous offerings of help and feel lifted and supported by the much available concern of others because you stop criticizing their imperfections, and stop pretending you don't need to change.

- With humility your confusion can turn into understanding because you allow yourself to be taught from many minds that are clear instead of trying to make sense with one mind that is ill.

- 有谦卑的态度，你的失望得以变成希望，因为你会开始信赖那些关心你并有能力提供帮助的人，而那些帮助是你自己永远找不到的。

是的，"征服谦卑之石"的确是开始走向通往平静生活的五块踏脚石之前，最重要的首要步骤。能做到"谦卑"，你就能相信别人，并有能力接受教导。当你可以去信赖，并能接受教导以后，就会发觉谦卑不但给你好处，更给你力量。换句话说，谦卑其实没什么好害怕的地方，或者会让你失去什么。我敢说如果你愿意研读这本书，而且已经读到这一页，那么你已经开始踏上谦卑之路了。恭喜你！

请将你对"征服谦卑之石"的想法与意见写在你自己的笔记本上。

- With humility your despair can turn into hope because you start to trust others who care for you and who are qualified to give you the assistance you could never find alone.

Yes, "conquering rock humility" is an essential prerequisite to starting the five step journey toward a more peaceful life. When you are humble, you are trusting and teachable. When you are trusting and teachable, you learn that humility gives you an advantage, and is a strength. In other words, there is really nothing to fear or to lose by becoming humble. My guess is if you are willing to read this book this far, you are already well on your way. Congratulations!

Please write notes and thoughts on "Conquer Rock Humility" in your notebook.

步骤一：察觉你的疾病

要察觉躁郁症这个刁滑的疾病的方法之一，就是注意朋友、家人，或其他常跟你在一起的人对你的看法与评论。对你有相当认识的人，会在你自认一切情绪都处于"正常"范围的时候，察觉你的精神状态实际上是过高（亢奋）或者过低（抑郁）。问题是他们很有可能只察觉到"表面症状"，而不能察觉该情绪的真正起因。为了察觉躁郁症，你必须先确认这些表面症状的成因究竟是来自躁狂症还是抑郁症。这里有个帮得上忙的小测试。

研读以下的句子，看看你能不能辨识别人说的这些现象究竟是躁狂症还是抑郁症。

- 为何你总是看起来很难过的样子？（虽然你并不觉得自己是这样。）

Step I：IDENTIFY YOUR ILLNESS

One way to identify the tricky illness, bipolar disorder, is to pay attention to the comments and observations friends, family and other people who are close to you make. People who know you well will recognize when your highs and lows cycle beyond your personal "normal." The problem is they will most likely only be able to see "surface symptoms" and not the true cause. In order to identify bipolar disorder you must determine whether the root cause or motivation of the surface symptoms is actually mania or depression. Here is a quick exercise to help. See if you can identify depression or mania from the following comments people observing surface symptoms might make：

- Why do you always look so sad? (Even though you don't really feel sad.)

- 你得听着音乐才能把日子过下去，是不是？
- 为什么你一直感到愧疚、罪恶或担心？
- 酒或毒品给你带来什么好处了吗？
- 你总是看起来很累。
- 你想太多了吧。
- 放轻松，你别那么紧张，想开点，让它去吧。
- 为什么你要随便乱花那么多钱？
- 你对你这个想法热衷过头了，别忘了吃饭照顾身体。
- 别在午夜打电话跟我谈你的钓鱼经好吗？上床睡觉吧。

- You can't function without your music can you?
- Why do you feel guilty or worried all the time?
- What benefit does your alcohol or drugs give you?
- You always look so tired.
- You think too much.
- You need to relax and unwind. Just chill and let it go.
- Why do you spend money so frivolously?
- You are way too excited about this idea of yours. Take time to eat.
- Don't call me in the middle of the night to talk about a fishing trip. Go to bed.

　　记住，每一个人在生活中都会有些轻微的躁狂跟抑郁症状，所以刚才这些话，完全没有躁郁症的人也一定听到过。不过另一方面，在情况极端时，前五个句子会从察觉抑郁症状的人们口中说出来；若听见的是后五句，则是因为他们察觉了躁狂的症状。请你想一想别人常对你说，但他们在平常或习惯上却不会对别人说的（带着类似评论性的）话，然后用自己的笔记本列下清单。你可能要先等一两个星期后才开始列下这张清单，这样你比较有办法做出更正确更仔细的观察。当人们对你说到类似的话的时候，问问他们有没有跟别人说同样的话。如果没有，问他们"为什么对我这样说？"你可以先从问他们"你刚才是开玩笑的，还是觉得真的是这样？"开始你们的讨论。

　　Remember, everyone suffers mild symptoms of mania and depression at different points in their lives. These comments could be made to people who don't have bipolar disorder. On the other hand, in the extreme, the first five comments could come from people observing depression. The last five could be made while observing mania. Take a minute and list comments people often make to you that you feel aren't "normal" or "typical" things they say to others, but could be observations of bipolar surface symptoms. You may want to wait a week or two before you start your list so you can have time to make a good, conscious observation. When people make the comments you write down, ask them if they make the same comments to others, and if not, why do they make them to you? Perhaps you could start the conversation by asking them, "Are you just saying that or are you serious?"

（如果你的个性比较内向、较少跟别人交流，或者你跟别人沟通的经验不是很多，又或是别人没有对你直接说出这些话，也许比较有效的办法是：你自己观察自己。你可以把清单的标题改成"我常重复的习惯、情绪和念头。"为了帮助自己知道写下什么东西，你要变得对自己在各种情形下做出的反应有警觉。问问自己："我承受压力的时候会做出什么事？""如果我开始心情沉闷，会有什么念头？""什么事情让我晚上睡不着？"等等。）

请将别人常对你说而你认为他们不太对别人这样说的（带有评论性质的）话写在自己的笔记本上。

（If you have a more introverted personality and don't talk or interact with other people very much, or if no one makes any significant comments to you, perhaps it would be more beneficial to make personal observations. You could change the title of your list to: "My recurring habits, emotions, and thoughts." To help yourself know what to write down, try to become aware to how you react to different situations. Ask yourself, "What do I do when I feel stressed?" "If I start to feel down, what thoughts come to my mind?" "What causes me to lose sleep at night?" etc.)

Please write common comments others make to you that you don't think they make to others in your notebook.

经过三四个星期的观察后，如果觉得你所写下的东西可能代表你有躁狂症和（或）抑郁症的话，应该把这份清单给社工、家庭医师或精神科医生看看。深入地谈谈你跟别人的谈话，以及他们对你说的那些（带有评论性质的）话或你对自己的观察。你可能会发现你原以为"不正常"的习惯、情感和思想其实正常得不得了，也可能发现你只不过需要一些心理辅导，或去找一堂"了解人类行为"的课来听听，或与医生做过更多讨论和检验后，他会确认你身体里有躁郁症存在。这种诊断结果使人惊讶，但如果发生了，试着把它想象成早期发现的癌症：虽然诊断结果吓人，但至少可以确定你已经趁这种疾病在你体内长成某些真正吓人的东西之前，早一步把它给揪出来了。

If after three or four weeks of observation you feel like the things you write down could be indicators of mania and/or depression, take the list to a social worker, family doctor, or psychiatrist. Discuss in depth the conversations you had with the people who made the comments, or the self evaluation you have done. You may find that your "not normal" habits, emotions and thoughts are all perfectly normal. You could discover that the only help you need is some counseling or an "Understanding Human Behavior" class. Or, after more sessions and tests, your doctor might identify bipolar disorder in you. This diagnosis can be shocking. But if it happens, think of it as you would an early discovery of cancer. It might be alarming to have in you, but at least you caught it early before it grew into something really scary.

　　无论如何，当你去找专业的建议时，要先在心理上做好"我要带着诊断的结果继续过日子"的准备。这样做，是通向更平安生活时必要的下一个步骤。

　　请将你对"察觉你的疾病"的想法与意见写在自己的笔记本上。

Whatever the case, when you seek a professional opinion, go prepared to authorize your diagnosis into your life. This will be the next necessary step toward a more peaceful life.

Please write notes and thoughts on "Identify Your Illness" in your notebook.

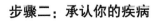
步骤二：承认你的疾病

你对自身疾病的态度，显示你是否接受标明"患了心理疾病的人"的标签。对某些人而言这件事情不难，但对另一部分人而言它可能是最困难的步骤。人们不愿承认自己生病的一些指标状况可能为：

- 否认。一直抱怨问题出在自己以外；或根本不愿意承认有什么问题。
- 对于任何想要帮助他的人发脾气。把生活中因疾病而发生的麻烦都归咎于当时情境，或归咎于周遭的人。
- 不愿意学习与使用医生开的药物，也不愿把持续定期用药当成责任。
- 不断执着于幻想和错误想法，认为"我知道真相。"

Step II: AUTHORIZE YOUR ILLNESS INTO YOUR LIFE

The attitude you take toward your illness will tell whether or not you accept the label as "someone with mental illness." For some this may be fairly easy. For others, it might the most difficult step of all. Some indicators of people who do not authorize their illness into their lives could be:

- Denial. Claiming everyone and everything else has the problem; or refusing to even acknowledge there is a problem.
- Lashing out at anyone who tries to help. Blaming difficulties associated with the illness on their situations in life, or other people in their lives.
- Unwillingness to learn about and take prescribed medications consistently and responsibly.
- Clinging to delusions and false ideas of "I'm the only one who knows what is really happening."

- 退出往常让他快乐的活动。
- 屈服于躁狂症和抑郁症所带来的怪念头，向人表示："我就是这样。如果爱我就要接受。"

不愿意承认在自身有疾病存在，只会延长自己（以及身边付出关怀的人）受折磨的时间。如果你发觉自己真的在做以上所写的事的话，问问你自己这个问题：要跌到多深，我才愿意开始"止跌回升"？这里有些激励人心的想法，会让你有办法扭转局势：

- 社会对患心理疾病的人的态度变得越来越好。大部分人听到有人患心理疾病的反应是关心和谅解，而非排斥与无知地批评。换句话说，在今天的世界里患心理疾病不是什么丢脸的事。

- Withdrawal from activities that used to bring pleasure.
- Giving in to all the whims of depression and mania claiming, "This is just me. Love me the way that I am."

Those who refuse to authorize their illness into their lives only prolong their own suffering (as well as the caring people around them). If you find yourself doing the items listed above, ask yourself this question: How low will I have to fall before I allow myself to start climbing? Here are some encouraging thoughts to help motivate you to change directions.

- The attitude of society toward mental illness is changing for the better. The response of most people toward those with mental illness is concern and understanding; not disgust and ignorant criticism. In other words, having a mental illness in today's world is nothing to be ashamed of.

- 你不孤单。每个人一生中遇到的人里面，大约有三分之一的人会经验到某种心理疾病。试试看这个主意：下次你跟邻居或朋友聊天的时候，告诉他你现在在读一本有关躁郁症的书，问他认不认识任何有心理疾病的人。我敢赌他或他认识的某人患了抑郁或其他心理疾病。

- 你能用电话或网络找到免费的协助团体。

- 每个人在今生都会面对疾病。当关心你的人发现你愿意诚实且开放地面对、承担自己的疾病时，你们之间的距离会拉得更近，因为在他们的眼里，你是一个真诚的人。

- You are not alone. During their lifetimes, one in three people will experience mental illness of some type. Try this experiment. The next time you're shooting the breeze with a close neighbor or friend, tell her you're reading a book about bipolar disorder. Ask her if she knows anyone who suffers from mental illness. Chances are or someone she knows has depression or some other type of mental illness.

- Free support groups are readily available with a simple phone call or internet search. (I recommend www. NAMI. org for those in the USA.)

- Everyone faces illness in this life. When others who care about you find out you are facing your illness with honesty and openness, it shortens distances between you and makes you seem like a "real person."

在生活中承认躁郁症存在的意思，就是你可以对着镜子，真诚地微笑并毫不羞赧地对自己说："我是患了心理疾病的人，而且我知道这没啥大不了。"在你心里给这种态度留下一席之地，可以帮助你睁开眼睛，并使你看到其他人也艰辛地背负着他们生活中的种种难处。承认躁郁症的存在能为你带来正确的思想与态度，好让你从疾病带来的困难和挑战里得到学习并且成长，也可以为你身边想给你提供帮助的人打开一扇门。承认在你的生活中确实存在躁郁症，你会停止用责怪的眼光往外看，开始朝自己心里面搜寻自我提升的方法。你也会开始发觉疾病跟你的生活方式、习惯，甚至与你的人格个性都交缠在一起。了解到这点后，你应该会从心里渴望学习并了解所有有关你疾病的事——还有你自己。然后你会到达下一块踏脚石：明白。

请将你对"承认你的疾病"的想法与意见写在自己的笔记本上。

Authorizing bipolar disorder into your life means you can look into the mirror with an honest smile and without any shame as you say the words, "I am a person with mental illness and I know it's no big deal." Allowing this authorization to take place in you can open your eyes and allow you to see others struggling to bear their crosses in life. Authorizing bipolar disorder into your life can give you the right mindset and attitude to actually learn and grow from the trials associated with the illness. It can also open the door to the available help around you. When you authorize your illness into your life you stop looking outward for blame and start looking inward for ways to improve. You also start to discover how intertwined the illness has become with your lifestyle, habits, even your personality and character. At this point you will probably gain an honest desire to learn and understand everything you can about your illness…and yourself. This is your next step.

Please write notes and thoughts on "Authorize Your Illness Into Your Life" in your notebook.

步骤三：明白"你自己"与"疾病"

躁郁症常会跟人本来自我的个性、习惯和生活方式混在一起。为了使你和你的疾病之间能分个明白，你必须要退一步，从外面朝自己心里面观察——好像朝清澈水面观看自己的倒影一样。用这种客观角度研究过去的种种，可以帮助你看到你的个性在什么时候开始被躁郁症混入。下面这几点，列出人格开始与躁郁症混合时经常会表现出来的行为和思维。

- 小看自己。"我一定是个失败者，因为当别人高兴的时候，我却感到闷闷不乐。"（抑郁症状）

- 激昂无比。感觉自己高人一等，比他人更特别、更火热、更浪漫、更有特权或受神钟爱，或比别人多话、心智比别人更敏锐聪明。（躁狂症状）

Step III：UNDERSTAND YOUR ILLNESS & YOURSELF

Bipolar disorder has a tendency to mesh itself with a person's personality, habits, and lifestyle. In order to understand your illness and yourself, you have to step back and look at yourself from the outside in - as if you were looking at your reflection in a clear pool of water. Studying your past with this view can help you see when your personality started to become intertwined with bipolar disorder. Below is a list of common behaviors and thought processes that could indicate a tangle of personality and bipolar disorder.

- Lowered self esteem. "I must be a loser because I feel down when everyone else is happy." (depression)

- Grandiose feelings. Feeling higher, more special, more intense, more romantic, more privileged or in favor with God, having more to say, mentally sharper and brighter than everyone else. (mania)

- 完美主义。"我知道我在钢琴比赛上得到冠军，但那真是场很烂的演出。我弹错了两次！"很少能够接受"够好了"的评价。因为完美是唯一能接受的标准。（抑郁或躁狂症状）

- 强迫自己"应该"如何如何的想法。"我应该更快乐""我应该把事做到最好""我应该是个更好的人""我应该更努力工作"。（抑郁症状）

- 对过去无法释怀。"如果我能和她复合，那么我就可以再次像从前一样振奋。"（躁狂之后的抑郁症状）

- 悲观想法。"生命实在很没意思，我不如放弃尝试算了？"（抑郁症状）

- 执迷不悟：让某件事持续干扰你数个月甚至数年（躁狂症状）

- Perfectionism. "I know I took first place at the piano recital, but it was a horrible performance. I messed up two times!" Rarely able to accept praise or "well enough" because perfect is the only acceptable standard. (mania or depression)

- "I should be" thinking. "I should be happier;" "I should be the best at everything;" "I should be a better person;" "I should work harder." (depression)

- Hanging on to the past. "If I can just get back my girlfriend I'll feel high again." (depression following mania)

- Negative thinking. "Life just stinks. I might as well not even try." (depression)

- Obsession. Letting something bother you for months or years. "I just can't let it go." (mania)

其实要觉察出哪些性格表象来自躁郁症，哪些来自你生长的环境，哪些又是你本有的天性，这种事困难得几乎不可能。虽然如此，当你开始明白你自己和你的疾病时，为什么不把不好的性格特质归因于疾病，而把好的特质归因于原来的自己呢？照我的看法，我相信实际上好性格的特质就是真正的你，而不好的特质只不过是能治好的、能改变的疾病。现在，请你暂时向"后"退一小步，从远观的角度观察一下自己。

请利用自己的笔记本写出你性格特质当中好的部分，然后再写出不好的部分。

It's actually next to impossible to determine for certain which personality traits developed from the influence of bipolar disorder, which ones came from your upbringing, and which ones you were just born with. Still, as you begin to understand yourself and your illness, why not pin the bad traits on the illness and the good traits on yourself? I'm prone to believe that in actuality the positive traits are the real you and the negative traits are the treatable, changeable disorder. Take a minute now to step back and look at yourself from a distance. In your personal notebook, list some of your positive personality traits, and then list some of your negative personality traits.

Please write your positive personality traits and your negative personality traits in your notebook.

　　当你写完这些特质，请按照你的判断，针对那些性格特质的来源写下"抑郁症状""躁狂症状"或者"真正的自我"。然后把这份结果拿给你的精神科医生、专业心理辅导，或你常见的医生看，跟他谈谈各种治疗的方法。当你明白如何分辨疾病和你自己时，你已经开始走向更平静生活的下一步：控制你的疾病。

　　请将你对"明白'你'与'疾病'"的想法与意见写在笔记本上。

After making your lists, go back and write either "depression," "mania," or "just me," depending on where you feel the traits came from. Show this list to your psychiatrist, professional counselor, or your family doctor. Discuss methods of available treatment. When you do this you are starting the next step toward a more peaceful life: taking control of your illness.

Please write notes and thoughts on "Understand Your Illness and Yourself" in your notebook.

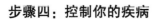

步骤四：控制你的疾病

明白自身患了躁郁症之后，往往使我们不得不认清一个难以接受的事实，那就是：它是一种慢性（持续性）的疾病。千万不要让这个信息使你窒息或放弃尝试。希望依然存在，得到躁郁症的人的确有办法去过有成就与快乐的生活。让你获胜的方法，就是控制你的疾病。虽然你无法阻断水流，但你却可以导引它的流向。也就是说，你可以从类似"我想要完全医好这个疾病"的态度改变为"我愿意学习带着躁郁症过好的生活"。下面是一些会帮你引导水流并学会控制的方法：

- 学习聆听身体传达给你的声音，留意那些能影响躁狂和忧郁症状强弱的事物。比如：深夜一边喝含咖啡因的饮料一边看电影，会不会使躁狂思想增强并让你睡不着觉？

Step IV：CONTROL YOUR ILLNESS

Understanding bipolar disorder often brings the hard realization that it is a chronic illness. Don't let this understanding choke you up or stop you from trying. There is hope. There is a way to live productively and pleasurably with bipolar disorder. The thing you can do to help is to take control. You can't stop the river, but you can direct its flow. This means changing your attitude from "I want this illness cured." to, "I will learn to live with my illness." Some things you can do to direct the river and take control are：

- Learn to listen to your body and recognize what influences the degree of depression and mania. For example：does watching late night movies while drinking caffeine drinks amplify your manic thinking and rob you of sleep?

- 在医生的指导之下，试着在日间、夜间不同的时间服药，留意什么时候用药效果最好。譬如，如果早上是抑郁症状的最高潮，那么或许早上就是使用抗抑郁药的最佳时机。
- 学习去察觉那些使你失去宝贵睡眠的躁狂式思维，找出反抗它们的办法，比如研读一本可以让你放轻松的书。
- 学习去察觉那些让你抑郁的念头，并以乐观的想法取代它。我建议你去想一些使人振奋的歌词与音乐。

- Under the direction of your doctor try taking your medications at different times of the day or night to find the best results. For example：if depression hits you hardest in the morning, perhaps that would be the best time to take your antidepressant medication.
- Learn to recognize manic thoughts that steal precious sleep. Find a way to counter them such as reading a relaxing book.
- Learn to recognize depressive thoughts and counter them with positive uplifting ones. I recommend thinking of lyrics and tunes of uplifting music.

- 用"回想"的方法，将所有负面、漫无头绪、极端的思想以务实、乐观的思想取代之。譬如："为什么那时抑郁症状突然出现呢？嗯，因为我失去生命中最好的情人，我想我永远不会结婚。为何我开始有这种感觉呢？因为我的脑海里有一首悲哀的乡村音乐回荡着。我在哪儿听到这首悲哀的歌呢？噢！我想到了，是我去购物的店里所放的音乐。我能做什么事情来控制这个让我抑郁的想法呢？我知道虽然不可能挽回女友，但我可以在今晚的舞会上邀请另外的女孩与我共舞。"

请用自己的笔记本写下一些可以帮你控制疾病的点子。

- Use "thought backtracking" to replace negative, all – encompassing, extreme thoughts with realistic, positive ones. For example: "Why has depression suddenly hit me? Well, I feel like since I lost the love of my life, I will never get married. How did I start feeling that way? I had a sad, country song in my head. Where did I hear the sad country song? Oh yeah, they were playing it in the store where I was shopping. What can I do to take control of this depressing thought? I can understand that although I can't bring my girlfriend back, I can go to the dance this Friday night and ask a different girl to dance with me."

Please write notes and thoughts on "Ideas to Take Control of My Illness" in your notebook.

步骤五：提升你的生活

抑郁症状会让你以为梦想只能在你睡着时才会成真，躁狂症状则会告诉你梦想就在你脚下；然而真理会帮你知道：抑郁症状只是一片掩盖你梦想的乌云，而躁狂症状是一种只要好好控制，反而可以帮你实现梦想的东西。当你尽力去察觉、承认、明白，还有控制好你的躁郁症时，你最后会发现你立足在更高的地势上。若你抬起头来环顾周围，你会开始看到许多使你梦想成真的机会。

在自己的笔记本上，请用几分钟写下你的梦想，即使它们已被乌云盖住了很多年。

Step Ⅴ：HEIGHTEN YOUR LIFE

Depression would have you believe that dreams only happen when you are sleeping. Mania will tell you that dreams are beneath you. Truth will tell you depression is only a cloud cover that hides your dreams, and mania is a power that, when controlled, can actually help you achieve them. As you work hard to identify, authorize, understand, and control your bipolar disorder you eventually will find yourself standing on higher ground. If you lift up your chin and look around, you will start to see opportunities for your dreams to come true.

Please take a minute and in your notebook write down your dreams even if they have been clouded over for years.

再检视一遍你刚刚罗列的梦想，在每个梦想边写上"幻想"或"实际"。当我们在头脑里架构梦想，并试着让它们在现实生活里实现的时候，很重要的问题是：这些梦想只是幻想，还是它们够实际？幻想是骗子，它会告诉你不用尽力追逐梦想就会达成，并且"从此过着幸福快乐的生活。"幻想通常虚假——它们无法真正抓在手里，而且不可能成功。幻想型的梦想会这样说："也许有一天你真能那么幸运。"

在另一方面，实际型的梦想则是从小地方开始，一步一步以小成果为基础建立起来，直到伟大的理想实现。你可以构筑合理、可行的计划来达成实际型的梦想，并且，你为了让成果继续维持，即使达成理想，你仍必须继续付出努力。

以下，是一些实际型梦想的范例，可以帮你思考和记住你的实际型梦想。

- 重新申请接受高等教育——即使当个兼职学生——而且耐心读到毕业。

Now look back at your list and by each dream write whether it is a "fantacy" or "reality" dream. When thinking about dreams and trying to have them happen in life, it's important to ask the question, "Are my dreams fantasy or reality?" Fantasy is a deceiver. It tells you that you can obtain your dreams without effort and keep them "happily ever after." Fantasy dreams are really only illusions without substance and impossible to achieve. Fantasy dreams say, "Maybe someday I'll be lucky and get it." Reality dreams, on the other hand, start small and build on each other to become something great. You can make reasonable, doable plans to achieve reality dreams. And, when you achieve reality dreams you have to work to keep them alive. Listed below are some examples of reality dreams to help you think about and remember your reality dreams.

- Reenrolling in higher education – even if it's just part time – and working patiently toward graduation.

- 再次去约会，这次我知道我的心理疾病已得到治疗，而且我有能力建造一个正常的家庭生活。
- 永远记住哪些人在我的生活里是最重要的，并以此控制急躁的表面症状。
- 用每周五天的慢跑来增加我的体力，直到我能参加 10 公里的比赛。

留意每个梦想是如何一步一步实现的，还有它们完成时如何打开下一道更远大梦想的门。现在你已知道幻想型和实际型的梦想的差别，请你再次回顾你所写下的梦想，并选出一个实际型的梦想来（如果没写到实际型梦想的话，可以重新思索一个）。

- Starting to date again, this time with the knowledge that my mental illness is being treated and a normal family life is possible for me to achieve.
- Controlling the surface symptom of irritability by remembering who is most important to me.
- Building up my stamina by jogging five times a week until I am in shape enough to run a 10km road race.

Notice how each dream can be worked up to, and how achieving them opens the door for new, higher dreams. Now, you understand the difference between fantasy and reality, look back at your list of dreams and choose one of your reality dreams (if you didn't write one down, think about and find a reality dream in your mind).

　　利用自己的笔记本写下让你能做出计划的具体步骤，然后朝着计划前进，去达成它，让这个梦想成为未来的你的基础。记住，最后的步骤不是完成你的梦想，而是用你的梦想提升你的生活，让你可以发展其他更远大的梦想。

　　请将帮助你实现"实际型"梦想的可行步骤写在自己的笔记本上。

In your notebook, please write specific steps you can take to plan for, work toward, achieve, and then to build on your reality dream. Notice the last step isn't to achieve your dream, it is to use your dream to heighten your life and build you up toward other dreams.

Please write in your notebook steps you can take to achieve your reality dreams.

当你去计划并朝着目标努力，进而完成梦想的时候，你会用感激的态度来珍惜这段经验。你同时也会感激那些鼓励和帮助你的人。实现你的梦想，并且看到其他梦想在它上面继续建立起来，真是个奇迹般的经验。然而，毕竟这一切：察觉→承认→明白，进而控制疾病，不正是一段请求并接受他人对你的帮助的过程吗？是的，这是一个奇迹！看看你现在的生活，你虽然还没得到完美的治疗，但你的确找到了更平静的生活。

请将你对"提升你的生活"的想法与意见写在自己的笔记本上。

When you plan for, work toward, and achieve your dreams, you cherish them with a grateful heart. You also appreciate others who offered encouragement and assistance while you worked toward your dreams. Achieving your reality dreams and seeing them build on each other is a miraculous experience. But, after all, wasn't part of the process of identifying, authorizing, understanding, and controlling your illness enlisting and accepting help from others? Yes, it's a miracle! Look at your life now. You haven't reached perfect healing, but you have found a more peaceful life.

Please write notes and thoughts on "Heighten Your Life" in your notebook.

第八章　写给病患的照顾者、家人及朋友

先决条件：征服谦卑之石

身为照顾者，也许你所面临最困难的一件事，就是你非常渴望去帮助你所爱的、患了躁郁症的亲友，但他不欢迎你的帮助，甚至会把你赶走，或不客气地叫你闪远一点。看到他（们）独自在另一个拒绝你进入的世界里痛苦地承受着一切，实在令你心碎。要如何才能让他们知道：只要愿意敞开心扉让你参与其中，他们所需的帮助是无处不在的？

Chapter 8
For Caregivers, Family and Friends

Prerequisite：CONQUER ROCK HUMILITY

Perhaps the most difficult thing you face as a caregiver is yearning to help your loved ones who suffer with bipolar disorder, but instead of welcoming assistance, they push (or shove) you away. It breaks your heart to see them suffer all alone in a world that they refuse to let you into. How can you make them know that help is all around if they will just open their hearts and let you in?

关于这个问题，我的答案并不是我喜欢的那种安慰式的说法，但我觉得它才是真理——你唯一也是最应该做的事，就是先保重自己的身心健康与安全，第二件事则是为你所爱的人耐心祈祷，祈求他会找到并爬上"谦卑之石"。爬上谦卑之石意味着他选择用这个态度来面对他的问题：

"我需要帮助；我有弱点；我愿意听别人的话而改变我自己。"

The answer I give to this question is not as comforting as I would like it to be, but I feel it is the truth. The best you can do is to first, protect your own health and safety, and second, pray patiently for your loved ones that they will find and conquer "rock humility." Conquering rock humility means they choose to embrace the words and attitude of：

"I need help; I have weakness; I am willing to listen to others and change myself."

虽然你所爱的人必须单独去寻找谦卑之心，但根据我自己的经验，（旁人的）爱心跟耐心可以帮助并鼓励他较快找到；强横的逼迫或尖锐的批评通常只会让他们更硬起心来反抗。除此之外，一个好榜样也是很有效的助力——即使你认为你自己没有任何需要改变或改进的地方，但如果你所爱的人（病患）看见连你都愿意谦卑、甘于改变自己以获得更好的生活，也许他们会更有意愿去跟随你的脚步，进而改变他们自己。

无论用什么方法，他们只有在找到并爬上谦卑之石后，才能够和你一同开始，为迎向更平静的生活走出第一步：察觉疾病。

请将你对"征服谦卑之石"的想法与意见写在笔记本上。

Although humility is something your loved ones must find alone, my experience is that love and patience can help encourage it to come sooner, while overbearing force and hard-voiced criticism usually only hardens their resistance. I also know that example is a powerful force. Even if you don't think you have areas that need change and improvement, perhaps if your loved ones see you humble yourself and be willing to change your life for the better, maybe then they will be more prone to follow your lead and do the same for themselves. However it comes, only after they find and conquer rock humility can they start working with you on the first step toward a more peaceful life: Identifying the illness.

Please write notes and thoughts on "Conquer Rock Humility" in your notebook.

第一步　察觉你（所爱的人）的疾病

要帮助你尽早察觉所爱的人得了躁郁症有个好方法，就是透过观察其"表面症状"来辨识真正的病因究竟是抑郁或是躁狂症，这个方式并不像通常所说的那么简单。首先，即使是精神正常的人，也都会有兴奋与沉闷的起伏感受；其次，那些看起来异于常人的行为或许是受到躁郁症以外的因素影响所致。然而，察觉最根本的原因，是开始了解你所要面对的是什么，该如何去帮助对方的最好方法。如何透过表面症状来治疗或处理病因，你应该已经略知一二。以下是一些例子：

- 你让四岁的女儿在晚上看一部电影，以至于她在平常上床睡觉的时间仍然醒着；当电影结束，你告诉她该是关上电视、上床睡觉的时候，她开始大哭大闹。

Step I：IDENTIFY YOUR（LOVED ONE'S）ILLNESS

A good way to help identify bipolar disorder early in your loved one's life is tolook past surface symptoms and recognize the real cause：depression and/or mania. This is not as easy as it sounds because, first of all, even healthy people experience mild highs and lows. Second, the behavior that seems out of the ordinary may be influenced by something other than bipolar disorder. Still, identifying the root cause, whatever it may be, is the best way to begin to understand what you are dealing with and how to help. You probably already know a little about looking past surface symptoms and treating the root cause. Here are some examples：

- After letting your four year daughter stay up way past her bed time to watch a movie, when you tell her it's time to turn off the TV and go to bed, she starts fussing and throwing a nasty fit.

她尖叫着说她想看另一部电影，但你没有允许，因为你知道她哭的真正原因是她已经累了，而不是真的需要看另一部电影。跟她讲道理是徒然无功的，所以你只好把她抱起来，带她回到她房间的床上。虽然在回房的过程中她不断踢腿抗拒，但当她被放在床上时，她几乎立刻就睡着了。

- 每次到高海拔的山地去钓鱼时，你都有偏头痛发作的毛病。所以你在前次露营的时候吃了止痛药，药效能稍微缓解一下你的不适，但当药效消失，偏头痛总是会再度发作。最后，在你自我检查、接受医生的咨询之后，你终于发觉偏头痛的真正原因是饥饿，以及不规律的排泄所致。

She screams that she needs to watch another movie. You don't allow it because you know the real reason she is crying is because she is tired, not that she needs to watch another movie. Trying to reason with her is impossible so you pick her up and carry her to bed. Although she kicks and fights all the way to the bedroom, after lying down she almost immediately falls asleep.

- Every time you go on trout fishing outings in high elevation mountains you always develop a migraine headache. On previous camps you took pain medication which helped for a while but when it wore off the headache always returned. Finally, after a self examination and a consultation session with a doctor, you learn that the real reason for your headache is due to an empty stomach and irregular bowel movements.

　　于是在下一次去高山钓鱼的时候，你选择不吃止痛药，宁可花时间好好吃东西，并在需要的时候就乖乖去上厕所。结果，你的头痛问题就像营火的灰烟一样，完全消失不见了。

　　如果那位在哭闹的小女孩的父母让她再看另一部电影，会发生什么事呢？如果那位高山钓客在每次感到头痛时，就大口吞下阿司匹林呢？问题反而有越来越严重的可能。在很多时候，当所爱的人开始受躁郁症影响而发生某些行为（表面症状）的时候，照顾者反而看不见那个"很累的孩子"（抑郁症），或是那"饿得咕咕叫的肚子"（躁狂症）才是最根本的问题所在，因此他们只能试着治疗他们所看到的表面症状。因为没被察觉，真正的疾病将会悄悄地、持续地扩大，直到病患在某一天把生活搞得天翻地覆，精神崩溃终于发作。不要被躁郁症的表面症状蒙蔽了。

The next time you hit the mountains, instead of popping pain pills, you take time to eat well and sit well when needed. Like dissipating clouds of campfire smoke, the problem of the headache fades away into the thin air.

What would happen if the parents of the fussing child let her watch another movie? What would happen if the fisher just gulped aspirin every time he felt pain? Most likely, the problems would grow worse and worse. Very often, when a loved one begins suffering from bipolar disorder, caregivers can't see the "tired child," (depression) or the "hungry stomach" (mania) as the root cause. Thus, they only try to treat the surface symptoms they see. Unidentified, the real illness grows until life-shattering breakdowns occur. Don't be fooled by the surface symptoms of bipolar disorder.

给予你所爱的人足够的关心，才能够更加深入地观察和了解对方，以察觉进一步治疗患者真正的病因。以下是一些抑郁症患者可能会有的表面症状：

- 不健康的自我诊断：自行判断并使用其实对病情没有帮助的"药物"——包括会让人上瘾还有会使人自我毁灭的：酗酒，毒品（以及药物）滥用，未成年人接触色情内容（事实上所有年龄层都不应接触色情内容）等等。

- 还有一些感觉不太明显，且属于合法范围的自我处方"药物"：例如对音乐的上瘾或过度着迷、不断看电视或电影、花太多时间打电子游戏、太沉迷于上网，或过度睡眠。

Care enough to look deeper so you can identify and treat the true source. Some possible surface symptoms you may notice indicating depression could include：

- Unhealthy self medicating. These include the addictive and self-destructive "no nos:" alcohol abuse, drug abuse (illegal and prescription), and pornography for minors (Porn should be illegal for all ages!).

- Less obvious "legal" methods of self medication. These could include addictions or obsessions with music, constant TV or movie watching, too much time playing computer games, excessive internet surfing, or too much sleeping.

- 一直在烦恼：担心未来、担心身体健康、担心不存在或风险其实很小的问题，担心某一个人可能要死去……想烦恼的事太多，甚至会有无事担心时反而觉得不对劲的情况。
- 总是感到愧疚或有罪恶感：因为犯了小错，或因为和平凡人一样都有不完美的地方，总是感到自己不配进天国，对过去所犯的错无法释怀，也很难忘掉过去、展望未来。

这些例子乍看之下或许是彼此毫无关联的习惯、行为、想法和感受，但更仔细、更深入地看，每个表面症状都可能显示出抑郁症才是最根本的原因。你所爱的人采取的这些成瘾行为以及自我处方的"药物"，可能是他尝试着想逃脱因抑郁而来的痛苦和失望的方式，而种种担心或罪恶感，则可能是大脑曲解了身体总是沉重、郁闷的原因所致。

- Constant worry. Worrying about the future, worrying about health, worrying about nonexistent or low risk dangers, worrying that someone might die. Worrying so much that the person doesn't feel right if he doesn't have something to worry about.
- Constant guilt. Not feeling worthy of heaven due to small mistakes and normal human imperfections. Unable to let past mistakes go and move on.

All of these examples could appear to be habits, behaviors, thoughts, and feelings that are separate and unrelated. However, looking deeper than the surface may reveal depression to be the root cause for each one. The addictions and self medications could be attempts to escape depression's pain and despair. The worry or guilt could be the brain misinterpreting why the body always feels down.

有多少人借由各种表面症状来掩饰其患有抑郁症的事实，就可能有多少人罹患了躁郁症。请花几分钟，想想你所爱的人或正在照顾的病患，在自己的笔记本上，列出一些他或她的"表面症状"——就是那些看起来与一般人较不相同，而可能显示出抑郁症倾向的行为。

请将你所爱（或正在照顾）的人可能有抑郁症的表面症状写在自己的笔记本上。

就像地球有北极跟南极这两个极端一般，抑郁症的相对极端就是躁狂症。你可能会注意到的一些躁狂症的表面症状有：

- 脑中有些宏大的计划和过度夸张的想法，导致他/她饮食不正常且缺乏睡眠。

The number of surface symptoms disguising depression could be as varied as the number of people with bipolar disorder. Take a minute to think about your loved one, and then use the lines below to list some possible surface symptoms he or she has that seem "out of the norm." and may be indicating depression.

Possible Surface Symptoms of my Loved One that may Indicate Depression.

As north is to south, the opposite pole of depression is mania. Some of the surface symptoms you could notice include:

- Grandiose plans and over motivation leading to poor diet and lack of sleep.

- 他/她看起来过分的快乐，笑得太开心，而且认为这些脑袋发晕或过于开心快乐的状况带给他/她非常棒的感觉。
- 强势甚至有点霸道地与别人"分享"脑中的各种"创意点子"，往往会导致他人变得烦躁不耐、不愿妥协，或是强大的期望。
- "走火入魔"的执着：做大量且持续不停的艺术创作，或是急着要马上开始的百万富翁创业计划，清理或整理自己不满意的问题——即使之前已经花了很多时间做到非常枝微末节的地步。
- 因为思绪狂奔而睡不着。
- 强硬、不合理及不负责任地做决定。比如过度的消费、有外遇、赌博，或仅为了芝麻小事就辞掉工作。

- Being too happy, laughing too much, feeling too good to the point of giddy or over euphoric.
- Talking about ideas with overbearing intensity that often results in irritability and uncompromising, forceful expectations of others.
- Obsessions. Extensive art creation. Urgent "million dollar" business ideas that have to be acted upon right now. Spending hours cleaning or organizing to the point of not being satisfied even though hours of attention to extreme details has been made.
- Compulsive, irrational, and irresponsible decision making. For example spending money frivolously, having an affair, gambling, or quitting a job over what seems to be a petty issue.

就跟忧郁症的表面症状一样，躁狂症看来也能列出无尽的表面症状。

请在此花几分钟想一想，在自己的笔记本上写下你所爱（或正在照顾的）病患所做的，可能是躁狂症引起的表面症状。

现在，你已经写下了你的亲友（或受照顾者）可能因抑郁或躁狂症而引起的表面症状，请用温柔、体贴、没有批评且充满关爱的方式，与你的病患亲友在适当的时间谈谈你所写出的症状。请你们一起做，尝试去察觉这些表面症状的真正起因。刚开始，你的亲友可能完全不晓得为什么他会做出那些你所记叙的行为，你们也许要花很多时间深入地谈话，才能找寻到真正的原因。专业的心理咨询师拥有充分的学识和经验，可以教导并辅助你知道该如何做好这件事，或者也提供对你和你的亲人个别的心理咨询。

Just like the surface symptoms for depression, there could also be an endless list for mania.

Take a minute here to think about and list possible surface symptoms of mania exhibited by your loved one.

Now you have written down possible surface symptoms of depression and mania discuss your list with your loved one in a gentle, kind, non critical and caring way, and at a time that is appropriate. Together, try to identify the real cause for the surface symptoms. At first, your loved one may not know why he does the things you listed. It may take time to verbally dig to the true sources. Professional counselors have the education and experience to teach and coach you how to do it, or to have personal sessions with you and your loved one.

记得，从一开始就要采取正确的态度，表达出"我相信你可能是生病了，就像得了糖尿病或自闭症一样"的想法，这种态度会让你获得他/她的信任，而愿意让你带他/她去看心理顾问、医生，或精神科医师，以得到专业且准确的诊断。如果那些表面症状真的是因躁郁症而引起的，你接下来将要学习接受这疾病进入了你们的生活。这就是下一步骤：承认疾病。

请将你对"察觉你（所爱的人）疾病"的想法与意见写在自己的笔记本上。

As a start, remember, treating your loved one with the attitude of "I believe you could be ill just the same as if you had diabetes or autism." will allow you to gain the trust he needs to allow you to take him to a counselor, a doctor, or a psychiatrist for a professional and accurate diagnosis. If in fact the root cause of the surface symptoms turns out to be bipolar disorder, you will next need to authorize the illness into your lives. This is the next step.

Pleases write notes and thoughts on "Identify Your (Loved One's) Illness" in your notebook.

第二步：承认你（所爱的人）的疾病

世界的态度在改变。人们开始了解心理疾病只是脑部单纯的生理失常而已。但当这种病被诊断出的时候，病患还是可能感到羞惭甚至屈辱。在这种时候，你所爱的病患大概会突然变得敏感于人们透露出的"疯子""神经病""怪胎"一类对心理疾病轻率、不礼貌的话。如果病患像我一样，在自己小的时候曾不知不觉地对他人说过这样的话，就会感觉这些尖锐的话正冲着他们而来，直接针对他们的心射击。以下方法可以帮助你鼓励你所爱的患者如何在往后生活上承认他的疾病：

Step II：AUTHORIZE YOUR（LOVED ONE'S）ILLNESS INTO YOUR LIFE

The attitude of the world is changing. People are beginning to realize mental illness is simply a biological brain disorder. When the diagnosis is given, however, it still can be a very humbling, or even humiliating experience. At that point, your loved ones will probably suddenly become aware of every comment and every reference made toward crazies, loonies, freaks, weirdoes, whackos, and all the other mean and thoughtless references to the mentally ill. If they are like me, they probably used these words and jokes without thinking in their youth. Now, they feel like the words are being targeted, aimed, and fired straight at their hearts. Some things you can do to help encourage your loved one to authorize the illness into his or her life are：

- 承认你自己是心理疾病患者的家人或好友。不要对这个诊断结果否认、逃避或退缩。要面对它，要接受它。
- 当你跟别人谈你所爱的人生病的事时，不要在行为上表示羞耻，或在言谈中表现出尴尬的态度。相对的，你要用关爱、尊重，以及委婉诚实的方式来谈论，就像谈到某位患了糖尿病的人一样。
- 小心不要对你所爱的病患和所有其他患心理疾病的人开玩笑或讽刺。记住，也许你心里并没有把他们当作电视上的"神经怪胎"或是"街头疯子"，但你所爱的病患很可能把她自己看成这种人。
- 如果你所爱的病患针锋相对地抨击你的弱点时，要用耐心和理解的态度来包容他，不要试着反唇相讥。因为他的反应方式会强烈地受你的反应方式的影响。

- Authorize yourself as a family member or friend of a person with a mental illness. Don't deny, shun, or hide from the diagnosis. Face it. Accept it.
- Never act ashamed or embarrassed when talking to others about your mentally ill loved one. Instead, use kind, respectful, and tactful honesty. Speak about his illness the same way you would talk about someone with diabetes.
- Be careful not to joke, or make sarcastic comments, not just about your loved one, but about all mentally ill people. Remember, although you may not, she will probably put herself in the same category as "the crazy freaks on TV, or the loonies on the street."
- Be patient and understanding if your loved one lashes out, or starts pointing out your weaknesses whenever you try to talk about his.

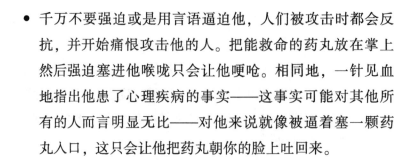

- 千万不要强迫或是用言语逼迫他，人们被攻击时都会反抗，并开始痛恨攻击他的人。把能救命的药丸放在掌上然后强迫塞进他喉咙只会让他哽呛。相同地，一针见血地指出他患了心理疾病的事实——这事实可能对其他所有的人而言明显无比——对他来说就像被逼着塞一颗药丸入口，这只会让他把药丸朝你的脸上吐回来。

- Never use brute or verbal force. People throw up resistance and build up resentment when they are attacked. Putting the lifesaving pill on your finger and shoving it down your loved one's throat would only make her choke. Likewise, although the blatant truth that your loved one is ill may be totally obvious to everyone else, verbally forcing this reality down her throat will most likely only cause her to throw it back up – right in your face.

在你所爱的人能承认他们是患了心理疾病的人以前，他可能会对每个人对他的看法非常敏感。有时候不说任何话可能跟说错话一样造成伤害，但你不必担心，知道该说什么与不说什么并不那么困难。你只要像在他们被诊断前那样爱他们和接受他们就好。这样简单的行为就是在告诉他们：承认得到躁郁症，不是什么羞耻或害怕的事。

请将你对"承认你（所爱的人）的疾病"的想法与意见写在自己的笔记本上。

Until your loved ones authorize themselves as people with mental illness, they will most likely be very sensitive of how others perceive them. Sometimes not saying anything can be just as damaging as saying the wrong thing. But don't worry. Knowing what to say and what not to say really isn't that big of a deal. Just treat them with the same love and acceptance that you did before the diagnosis. This simple act can show them that authorizing bipolar disorder into their lives is nothing to be ashamed or afraid of.

Please write notes and thoughts on "Authorize Your (Loved One's) Illness Into Your Life" in your notebook.

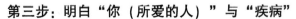

第三步：明白"你（所爱的人）"与"疾病"

身为一个照顾者，你可以在你所爱的人（病患）察觉他的疾病进入其生活之前，就开始进行"明白疾病"这一步骤。学习并理解在病患身上究竟会发生哪些情况，会是一个给予你慰藉的方式：一旦你明白了躁郁症，你就会知道它是可以治疗的。以下是一些你可以用来学习、明白躁郁症的资源：

- 网络。在网络上可以找到许多心理诊所，以及支持团。

Step III: UNDERSTAND YOUR (LOVED ONE'S) ILLNESS AND HIM/HERSELF

As a caregiver you can start the step of understanding the disorder even before your loved ones have authorized the illness into their lives. Learning what is happening to them can be a source of comfort because as you come to understand bipolar disorder, you learn that it is highly treatable. Following are some resources you can use to learn and understand bipolar disorder.

- The internet. There you can find many psychiatric clinics and support groups.

- 在你住家附近的图书馆：当你阅读图书馆的藏书时，要记住人们对心理疾病的了解才刚刚开始起步，那些 20 年前的书里宣告"没有希望""无药可医"，或"未知"的事情，可能在此刻已经是有希望的、可医治的，并获得越来越多深入的了解。

- 书店：在全世界，有许多私人出版社已经注意到人们对于心理疾病相关资讯的需求。因此，现今有越来越多以心理疾病为主题的出版物出现在市面上。

- Your local library. As you read books from the library remember that understanding of mental illness is still in its infancy. What may have been "hopeless," "untreatable," or "unknown" 20 years ago may now be hopeful, treatable and gaining more and more understanding.

- Your local bookstore. Private publishing companies all over the nation and world are recognizing the need and demand for information regarding mental illness. Consequently, more and more products (not just books) dealing with the subject of mental illness are coming available.

　　学习躁郁症的相关知识会帮助你开始了解，并分辨出你所爱的人与他所患的疾病之间的差异。我猜想你也将会证实你一直以来都相信的事实：你所爱的人是一个非常好的人，那些让他看来很奇怪、会冒犯人或是伤害自身的行为，都是来自一项相当具有挑战性的难缠疾病。在你运用前述所提供的资源，了解关于躁郁症的知识之后，请用几分钟的时间，回顾一下你所爱之人曾发生的事件和经验。写下你认为是被疾病所影响而引起的事件或对话，例如：在好几天偷偷不吃药后的某个失眠深夜里，我双眼发亮地告诉我妻子：只要人们有足够的信心，他们就能在天上飞，钱也会从树上自己长出来。

Learning about bipolar disorder will help you begin to understand the difference between your loved one and your loved one's illness. My guess is that you will discover confirmation of a truth you always believed in: your loved one is a good person whose seemingly strange, offensive, or self destructive thoughts and behavior stem from a challenging illness. After using the resources listed above to learn about bipolar disorder, take a minute to reflect back on incidents and experiences with your loved one. List the events or conversations that you believe were influenced or even controlled by your loved one's illness. For example: Late one sleepless night after a few days of secretly not taking my medication, with intensity in my eyes I told my wife people could fly and money could grow on trees if they had enough faith.

我的妻子没有对我的话大惊小怪，只是用全然理解的表情听我说话并点点头；她完全明白那是我的疾病在对她讲话，而不是真正的我。到了隔天早上，我发现我的药出现在浴室的洗手台上。

请将你所爱的人因受这可治疗的疾病影响或控制的事件写在笔记本上。

当你了解了躁郁症之后，你也会开始辨认出哪些事情是确实发生或没有发生在你所爱之人的身上。这可能会让你觉悟到，过去有很多时候你误会了你爱的人和他的疾病。请花点时间回想一下你曾与所爱之人发生的事件，并写下那些你所误会的事情。例如：当我的工作领导人看到了我因抑郁症而产生的表情时，他误以为我看起来很邪恶。

请将什么时候你误解了所爱之人的疾病写在笔记本上。

Instead of panicking, she just listened and nodded her head with the complete understanding she was just hearing my bipolar mania and not the real me. The next morning I found my pills sitting on the bathroom counter.

Please write past incidents you believe were influenced or controlled by your loved one's treatable illness in your notebook.

As you come to understand bipolar disorder you will start to be able to recognize what is really happening and what is not happening to your loved one. This may bring a realization that there have been times when you misunderstood your loved one and her illness. Take a minute to reflect on incidents you experienced with your loved one. Make a list of the times you misunderstood what happened. For example: When my employer saw my depression, he misunderstood it to be "a dark, evil countenance."

Please write down examples of times you misunderstood your loved one's illness.

现在，你已明了了躁郁症是如何影响一个人的行为与思想。请你想一想你那位患有躁郁症的亲人或好友，用你的理解之眼看着他（或是她），你所看到的难道不是一个非常优秀且不断对抗着难缠疾病的人吗？请花点时间，将你从所爱之人身上看到的优点都写下来。

请将你所爱之人拥有的优秀特质写在笔记本上。

Now you understand bipolar disorder and how it can influence a person's actions and thinking, think about your loved one. Looking at him or her with the eyes of understanding, don't you see a wonderful person battling a very challenging disorder? Take a minute and list the good traits you see in your loved one.

Please write the good characteristics of your loved one in your notebook.

如果你觉得对你所爱的人有帮助且感觉已到适当的时机，请把你写下的东西拿给你所爱的病患者看看。问问他是否同意你所写的内容，和他谈谈你所学习到的有关躁郁症的知识，以及你所知躁郁症会带给不同的人的影响。我相信让病患知道身为照顾者的你很在乎他、愿意尝试去了解他及他所经历的疾病，将会带给他们两方面的助益：第一，在他们了解自己疾病的过程中，他们可能会开始问你问题，将你视为资源，想借着你学习他们不知道的事；其次，在看到你为了明白他和他所患的疾病，而乐意付出关心的时候，他会因而受到鼓励而试图改变。

请将你对"明白"你（所爱的人）"与"疾病"的想法与意见写在自己的笔记本上。

If you feel it would be helpful and appropriate, show your lists to your loved ones. Ask them if they agree with what you have written down. Discuss with them the things you have learned about bipolar disorder and how it influences different people. I believe simply knowing you care enough to try and understand them and their illness can have a great influence on them for good in two ways. First, they may begin to ask you questions and start to draw on you as a source of information in their own process of coming to understand their illness. Second, seeing your willingness and caring effort to understand them and their illness may be the encouragement they need to find the courage and desire to start controlling their illness.

Please write notes and thoughts on "Understand Your (Loved One's) Illness and Him/Herself" in your notebook.

第四步：帮你所爱的人控制他/她的疾病

现在，我希望你和你所爱的人一起努力，好像团队一样。在你们开始"控制"这个新步骤时，身为照顾者的你最重要的事或许是"帮忙"而非"控制"。你若是担心太多而且太过于控制，可能对所爱的人的进步造成阻碍，甚至会使他开始退步。千万不要试着去控制你所爱的人，只是从旁协助。帮助你所爱的人控制躁郁症，需要耐心和开放式的沟通这两个基本要件，独断的强迫和竭力相抗则会损害他们。在你为了帮助你所爱的人控制他的躁郁症而研读以下建议的时候，请记住这个原则。

- 如果你所爱的人接受的话，跟他一起去看医生。

Step IV: HELP YOUR LOVED ONE CONTROL HIS/HER ILLNESS

Hopefully you and your loved one are working as a team by now. As you start this new step, perhaps the most important thing you as a caregiver can remember is the word "help" and not the word "control." Becoming too concerned and over controlling could ruin your loved one's progression and even set him or her back. Don't try to control your loved one. Instead, just offer help. Helping your loved one to control bipolar disorder takes patience and open communication. Brute force and power struggles destroy these elements. Keep this in mind as you read the list below of suggestions to *help* your loved one take control of his or her illness.

- If your loved one will let you, go to doctor visits together.

你能提供给医生一些你所爱之人没注意到的地方。看医生之前，先决定你们要一起去找医生还是轮流去，或一半一半，看哪种方法最好。有的病患不喜欢"秘密"，但也有的可能会受不了你给医生提出的报告。若决定一起去找医生，你与医生沟通时，也要体贴你所爱的人在一旁聆听的感觉。我身上有个例子：一回我跟妻子一起去找医生，虽然当她跟医生说明在我使用某种药物后产生易怒的副作用时我内心不太舒服，但听着她温柔的声音、体贴的口吻，我知道她并不是在批评我，只是诚实地告诉医生她所看到的事。

- 当你所爱的人换吃新药的时候，你可以每天帮她记下她的行为与情绪。有的药必须吃一个多月才能看出是否有效。

You can provide insight your loved one might not notice. Before the visit, decide whether it would be best to meet with the doctor together, separately, or both. Some patients don't like "secrets" while others might not want to hear your report to the doctor. When talking to the doctor together, be sensitive to the feelings of your loved one. For example: Although I felt irritated when my wife reported a certain medication made me irritable, her quiet, caring tone of voice let me know she wasn't being critical; she was only honestly reporting what she had observed.

- When experimenting with new meds keep a daily journal of your loved one's behavior and moods. Some medications take a whole month before they can be determined effective or not.

- 你所爱的人开始进步并朝好的方向改变的时候，要用赞美及乐观的鼓励帮助他获得成就感。留意并称赞你所爱的人，会帮助他知道你的确爱他，且是值得留在身边的伙伴。

躁郁症尤其是抑郁的部分往往让病患失去渴望培养与人们有恩爱关系。不过当他察觉、承认和明白疾病之后他/她又会发觉恩爱关系的重要。这个时候你可以鼓励他/她重心付出努力培养恩爱关系。按照我自身的经验，我知道如果你所爱的人能坚定地对重要家庭朋友的关系不断保持希望和努力的话，那么他就有办法控制他的疾病，重新找到通往梦想之路，并且过一种持续提升向上的生活。

请将你对"帮你所爱的人控制他／她的疾病"的想法与意见写在自己的笔记本上。

- Use praise and positive encouragement to help your loved one feel successful as he or she improves and makes changes for the better. Noticing and complimenting your loved one helps him or her to feel your love and realize even more that you are a teammate worth keeping.

Bipolar disorder, especially the depressive part, has a way of draining the desire to keep up loving relationships. However, when your loved one identifies, authorizes, and understands the illness, he/she will rediscover the importance of loving relationships. This is a good time to encourage your loved one to take efforts to regain loving relationships. My own experience is that doing so gives me the strength I need to move toward a heightened life.

Please write notes and thoughts on "Help Your Loved One to Control His/Her Illness" in your notebook.

第五步：提升你所爱的人的生活

"过向上提升的生活"意味着增进才能、拓展人生中的各种可能性，以及每天奋发不懈地面对挑战，追求生活中更大的幸福。简单来说，帮助你所爱的人"提升他的生活"的意思，就是鼓励他相信并追求"实际型"（可以一步步实现）的梦想。躁郁症，尤其抑郁症，就好像一片会把梦想盖住，甚至让人忘记曾有过梦想的巨大乌云。想想你所爱的人，然后写下你曾注意到的、他以前拥有过的梦想。

请将你所爱的人的梦想写在自己的笔记本上。

Step Ⅴ：HEIGHTEN YOUR（LOVED ONE'S）LIFE

Living a heightened life means increasing abilities, expanding possibilities, and rising up each day to the challenge of finding greater happiness in life. Simply put, helping your loved one live a heightened life means inspiring him to believe in and seek after realistic dreams. Bipolar disorder, especially depression, has a way of clouding out dreams and making the person forget she ever had them. Think of your loved one and list some dreams you have observed her to have earlier in life.

Please write some dreams of your loved one in your notebook.

现在看看你写的东西然后问自己："这些真的是我所爱的人他自己的梦想，还是我希望他拥有的梦想呢？"当我们鼓励所爱的人追求梦想的时候，很重要的一点就是：我们千万不要叫他去追求我们自己想要的期许和梦想。梦想应该是快乐的愿望，而且努力追寻的时候会变成一个让人满足、有成就感的好东西。下面，我列出那些爱我的人鼓励我去追求并达成我最大梦想时用过的几个方法。

- 用"允许事情自然发生"的方式来教导（别说："我不是早跟你说过事情会变成这样吗……"）。比如，有一晚我的躁狂症状来了，一个我自认为能赚大钱的"好主意"出现在我脑海里。我相信只要写一封简单的信，给制造篮球训练鞋的加挂附件（用绑在鞋上的特殊东西来训练人）公司的老板，可以让我马上有机会赚好几百万美元，而且会让我可以跳到足以把球灌进篮筐的高度。

Now look back at your list and ask yourself, "Are these really my loved one's dreams, or the dreams I wish she would want?" When encouraging loved ones to pursue dreams it is vital that we never force our own wishes and dreams on them. Dreams should be happy desires that, with effort, develop into something rewarding, positive, and worthwhile. Following is a list of things my loved ones did for me that encouraged me to pursue and achieve my best dreams.

- Allow natural consequences to do the preaching. For example: One night while on the manic side of the bipolar cycle, I came up with what I thought was a very "rich" idea. I believed a simple letter to the owner of a company who made attachments that strapped onto basketball training shoes would give me the opportunity to make millions and improve my vertical jump high enough to slam dunk a basketball.

当我给我的妻子看那封我那晚花了好几个小时写下的信，她并没有笑我，或批评我的新梦想。即使当我花了 50 美元买到那种运动鞋附件的时候，她也没讲任何怀疑或嘲笑的话。一个月之后，当我没有收到任何回信，而且没办法得心应手地用那个绑在鞋上的东西好好训练以致成效不彰的时候，这个天真的梦想自然也就放弃了。我的太太从来不需要说任何话，只是让这些梦想自然而然地消失。

When I showed my wife the letter I had spent much of the night writing, she didn't laugh or cut down my new dream. Even when I spent 50. 00 to purchase the shoe attachments she didn't criticize or express doubt. A month later when I received no return letter and was burned out and discouraged from inconsistent training and seemingly no results, I gave up on the dead-end dream. My wife never needed to say anything. She just let the dream go where it was meant to go.

- 要支持实际型的，甚至貌似简单的梦想。当我开始写鳟鱼诗的时候，我确定我家人那时的感觉也是：这只是个阶段性的，没有前景的梦想而已。虽然如此，他们还是支持着我，读我的诗，并给我一些建设性的建议和仁慈的赞美。他们的鼓励，帮我开始看见并相信一个新的梦想：当作家。从这小小的一步起，梦想开始一个叠一个地堆积起来。开始时不大，但我要"活出梦想"，我写作的能力进步了，我的作家之路拓展开了，而且当我看到自己的作品感动与帮助他人的时候，就越来越开心。这一切的开始，都源自于最初我想当作家的这个简单梦想，以及感受到被支持的缘故。

- Be supportive of the realistic and even seemingly simplistic dreams. When I first started writing fishing poetry I'm sure my family thought it was just a phase and not a dream with potential. Still, they supported me by reading my poems and offering genuine constructive suggestions and kind praise. Their encouragement helped me to see and believe in a new dream: becoming a published author. From that humble start the dreams started to build on each other. Starting small, but "living the dream," my writing abilities increased, my writing possibilities expanded, and I started to feel more and more happiness as my simple writing inspired and lifted others. All this came from simply feeling supported in my early writing dreams.

- 用温柔和爱心的方法指引你所爱的人朝向实际、可行的梦想。躁狂症思维的一个特色就是不着边际的幻想，而抑郁症思维的特色之一则是悲观和绝望。

虽然你已经帮助你所爱的人完成到目前为止的每一个步骤，但他追寻梦想时的思维习惯，可能还是需要你的帮忙与指引。以我为例，有一天晚上，当我在我父亲的建筑工地上了一整天辛苦的班之后，突然想到一个可以完全改善父亲公司经营的方法。我父亲身为老板，我想他完全可以因为我对管理和生意一窍不通，给我来一段长篇大论的"教训"。但他并没有这样做。而是请我到他的办公室去，为我解释什么事能改，什么事不能改。他用稳定、温柔的语气与我说话，指引我去思索一个不同的梦想——就是完成我的教育。

- Use gentle and loving persuasion to steer your loved one toward realistic and positive dreams. One of the characteristics of mania is grandiose thinking. One of the characteristics of depression is negative and despairing thinking.

Although you have helped your loved one to achieve each step up to this point, some of the thinking habits, when it comes to pursuing dreams, may still need your help and direction. For example, one night after a tough day at work as a laborer on one of my father's construction sites, I came up with a plan to completely redesign the management structure of his company. With my dad as the boss, I'm sure he could have really lectured me on how little I knew about management and business, but he didn't. Instead he called me in and explained the "can's" and "cant's" of the business. His kind-but-firm direction steered me toward a different dream of finishing my education.

　　相信你所爱的人的"实际型"梦想可以带领他到他从来没想过的高度。当你们开始踏上帮你所爱的人找到更平静生活的五个步骤之路时，他可能没想到这种不断向上提升的生活是可以做到的。我希望，并渴望在这个过程中你所爱的人会更加认识你，并学习到珍惜、尊敬你的爱和友谊。毕竟，若生活提升的结果只是让一个人过得比另一个人好，那有什么好处呢？我相信，当你们一起努力去"察觉""承认""明白"并"控制"你所爱的人的疾病的时候，你们两人都会发现生活不仅"提升"了，也更加平静了。

　　请将你对"提升你（所爱的人）的生活"的想法与意见写在自己的笔记本上。

Believing in your loved ones' realistic dreams can lead them to heights they probably never thought would be possible. When you first started the path of the five steps to help your loved ones find a more peaceful life, they probably never would have believed such a heightened life could be possible. My hope and desire is that along the way your loved ones discovered you and learned to cherish and respect your love and friendship. After all, what good is a heightened life if one person is above the other? I believe as both people work together to identify, authorize, understand, and control your loved ones' bipolar disorder, both of you will find your lives heightened and more peaceful.

Please write notes and thoughts on "Heighten Your (Loved One's) Life" in your notebook.